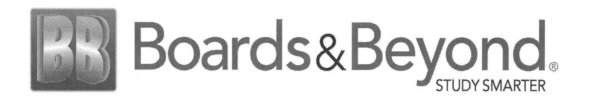

Boards & Beyond:
Immunology Slides

Color slides for USMLE Step 1 preparation
from the Boards and Beyond Website

Jason Ryan, MD, MPH

2022 Edition

Boards & Beyond provides a virtual medical school curriculm used
by students around the globe to supplement their education and
prepare for board exams such as USMLE Step 1.

This book of slides is intended as a companion to the videos for
easy reference and note-taking. Videos are subject to change
without notice. PDF versions of all color books are available via the
website as part of membership.

Visit www.boardsbeyond.com to learn more.

Table of Contents

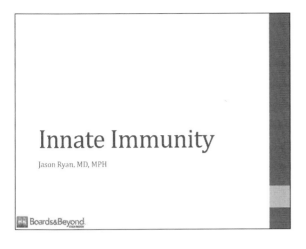

Innate Immunity

Jason Ryan, MD, MPH

Boards&Beyond

Barriers to Infection

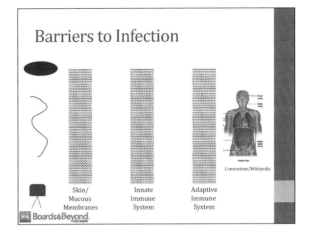

Skin/ Mucous Membranes · Innate Immune System · Adaptive Immune System

Connexions/Wikipedia

Boards&Beyond

Immune Systems

Innate	Adaptive
• Fast-acting system	• Slow-acting (days)
• Non-specific reaction	• Highly specific
• Same cells, same reaction to many invaders	• Unique cells activated to respond to a single invader
• No memory	• Memory
• 2nd infection same response as 1st infection	• 2nd infection: faster response

Boards&Beyond

Antigen Presentation

- Innate system can be activated by "free" antigen
  - Pathogenic molecules detected freely in blood, tissue
- Adaptive system requires "antigen presentation"
  - Pathogens must be engulfed by cells, broken down
  - Pieces of protein transported to surface
  - Antigen "presented" to T-cells for activation

Boards&Beyond

Cytokines

- Cell signaling proteins
- Often released by immune cells
- Stimulate inflammatory response
- Various subsets
  - Chemokine: Attracts immune cells (chemotaxis)
  - Interleukins: IL-1, IL,2, etc
  - Tumor necrosis factor (TNF): Can cause tumor death
  - Transforming growth factor (TGF)
  - Interferons: Named for interfering with viral replication

Boards&Beyond

Cluster of Differentiation (CD)

- Cellular surface molecules
  - CD3, CD4, CD8
- Found on many immune cells (T-cells, B-cells)
- Used to identify cell types
- Some used as receptor/cell binding

Boards&Beyond

Innate Immune System

- Phagocytes
  - Macrophages (hallmark cell)
  - Neutrophils
- Complement
- Natural Killer Cells
- Eosinophils
- Mast cells and Basophils

Innate Immunity
General Principles

- Recognize molecules that are "foreign"
- "Pathogen-associated molecular patterns" (PAMPs)
  - Present on many microbes
  - Not present on human cells
- Pattern recognition receptors
- Key receptor class: "Toll-like receptors" (TLRs)
  - Macrophages, dendritic cells, mast cells
  - Recognize PAMPs → secrete cytokines

Innate Immunity
Pattern Recognition

- Endotoxin (LPS)
  - LPS binds LPS-binding protein (found in plasma)
  - Binds **CD14 on Macrophages**
  - Triggers TLR4
  - Cytokine production: IL-1, IL-6, IL-8, TNF
- Peptidoglycan cell wall
  - NOD receptors (intracellular)
  - Nucleotide-binding oligomerization domain
  - Cytokine expression

Innate Immunity
Pattern Recognition

- Mannose (polysaccharide on bacteria/yeast)
  - Mannose-binding lectin (MBL) from liver
  - Activates lectin pathway of complement activation
- Lipoteichoic acid on Gram-positive bacteria
- Double stranded RNA
- Unmethylated DNA

Monocytes and Macrophages

- Macrophages: guardians of innate immunity
- Produced in bone marrow as monocytes
- Circulate in blood ~3 days
- Enter tissues → macrophages
  - Kupffer cells (liver)
  - Microglia (CNS)
  - Osteoclasts (bone)

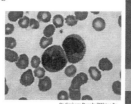

Dr Graham Beards/Wikipedia

Monocytes and Macrophages

- Three key functions:
  - Phagocytosis
  - Cytokine production
  - Antigen presentation

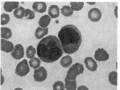

Dr Graham Beards/Wikipedia

Phagocytosis

- Macrophages engulf pathogens into phagosome
- Phagosome merges with lysosome
- Lysosomes contain deadly enzymes
- Death of bacteria, viruses

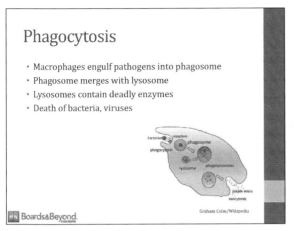

Graham Colm/Wikipedia

Phagocytosis

- Reactive oxygen species (superoxides)
  - Produced by NADPH Oxidase (respiratory burst)
  - Generate hydrogen peroxide H2O2 and O_2^-
- Reactive nitrogen intermediates
  - NO (nitric oxide) + O_2^- (superoxide) → $ONOO^-$ (peroxynitrite)
- Enzymes:
  - Proteases
  - Nucleases
  - Lysozymes (hydrolyze peptidoglycans)

Lysosome Enzyme Secretion

Lung Abscess

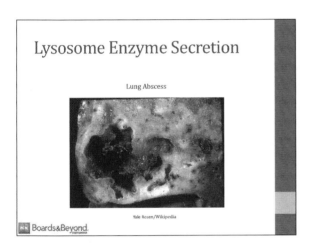

Yale Rosen/Wikipedia

Phagocytosis

- Some pathogens block this process
  - Tuberculosis modifies phagosome
  - Unable to fuse with lysosome
  - Proliferation inside macrophages
  - Protection from antibodies
- Chediak-Higashi Syndrome
  - Immune deficiency syndrome
  - Failure of lysosomes to fuse with phagosomes
  - Recurrent bacterial infections

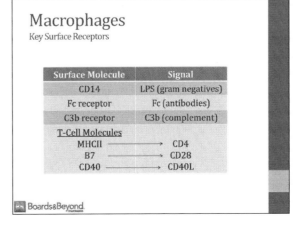

CDC/Public Domain/Wikipedia

Macrophages

- Macrophages can exist in several "states"
- Resting: Debris removal
- Activated ("primed"): more effective
- Major activators (via surface TLRs):
  - LPS from bacteria
  - Peptidoglycan
  - Bacterial DNA (no methylation)
- Also, **IFN-γ** from T-cells, NKC
- Attracted by C5a (complement)

Macrophages
Key Surface Receptors

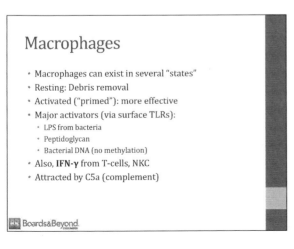

Surface Molecule	Signal
CD14	LPS (gram negatives)
Fc receptor	Fc (antibodies)
C3b receptor	C3b (complement)
T-Cell Molecules	
MHCII →	CD4
B7 →	CD28
CD40 →	CD40L

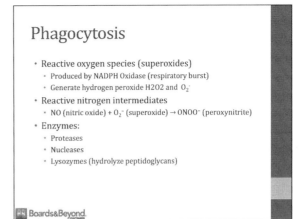
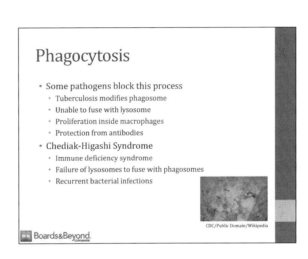

Macrophages
Cytokines

* Key cytokines are IL-1 and TNF-α
* Others: IL-6, IL-8, IL-12

IL-1 and TNF-α

* Both ↑synthesis endothelial adhesion molecules
    * Allows neutrophils to enter inflamed tissue
* IL-1
    * "Endogenous pyrogen" (causes fever)
    * Acts on hypothalamus
* TNF-α
    * Can cause vascular leak, septic shock
    * "Cachectin:" Inhibits lipoprotein lipase in fat tissue
    * Reduces utilization of fatty acids → cachexia
    * Kills tumors in animals ("tumor necrosis factor")
    * Can cause intravascular coagulation → DIC

IL-6, IL-8, IL-12

* IL-6
    * Fever
    * Stimulates acute phase protein production in liver (CRP)
* IL-8
    * Attracts neutrophils
* IL-12
    * Promotes Th1 development (cell-mediated response)

Neutrophil

* Derived from bone marrow
* Granules stain pink with Wright stain
    * Eosinophils=red, Basophils=blue
* Circulate ~5 days and die unless activated
* Drawn from blood stream to sites of inflammation
* Enter tissues: Phagocytosis
    * Granules are lysosomes (bactericidal enzymes)
* Provide extra support to macrophages

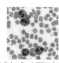

Dr Graham Beards/Wikipedia

Neutrophil
Blood stream exit

* Rolling
    * Selectin ligand neutrophils (Sialyl-Lewis X)
    * Binds E-selectin or P-selectin endothelial cells
* Crawling (tight binding)
    * Neutrophils express integrin
    * Bind ICAM on endothelial cells
* Transmigration
    * Neutrophils bind **PECAM-1** between endothelial cells
* Migration to site of inflammation
    * Chemokines: C5a, IL-8

Neutrophil
Blood stream exit

PMN

SL

Selectin

Step 1:
IL-1 and TNF stimulate expression selectin
PMNs bind selectin via selectin ligand

Neutrophil
Blood stream exit

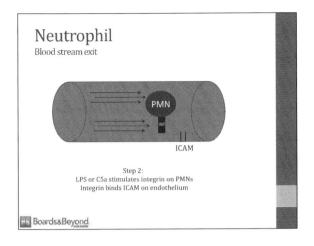

Step 2:
LPS or C5a stimulates integrin on PMNs
Integrin binds ICAM on endothelium

Neutrophils

- Small granules (specific or secondary)
  - Alkaline phosphatase, collagenase, lysozyme, lactoferrin
  - Fuse with phagosomes → kill pathogens
  - Also can be released in extracellular space
- Larger (azurophilic or primary)
  - Acid phosphatase, myeloperoxidase
  - Fuse with phagosomes only
- Band forms
  - Immature neutrophils
  - Seen in bacterial infections
  - "Left shift"

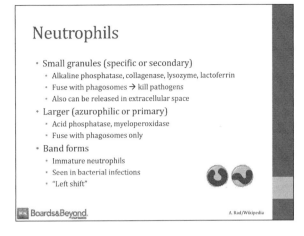

A. Rad/Wikipedia

Neutrophil

- Do not present antigen
  - Phagocytosis only
  - Contrast with macrophages: APCs and phagocytes
- Chemotaxins (attracters of neutrophils)
  - IL-8 (from macrophages)
  - C5a
- Opsonin: IgG (only antibody that binds neutrophils)

Complement

- Complement proteins produced by liver
- Most abundant is C3
- Frequent, spontaneous conversion C3 → C3b
- C3b binds amino and hydroxyl groups
  - Commonly found on surface of pathogens
- Failure of C3b to bind leads to rapid destruction

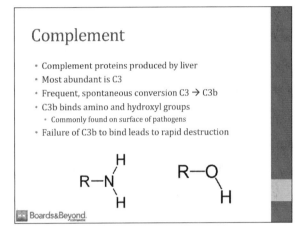

Complement

- C3b → MAC formation
  - Membrane attack complex
- Forms pores in bacteria leading to cell death

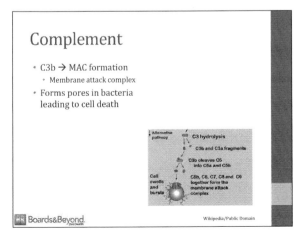

Wikipedia/Public Domain

Natural Killer Cells

- Two key roles:
  - Kill human cells infected by viruses
  - Produce IFN-γ to activates macrophages

Natural Killer Cells

- MHC Class I
  - Surface molecule of most human cells
  - Presents antigen to CD8 T-cells
  - Activates adaptive immunity against intracellular pathogens
- Some viruses block MHC class I
- NKC destroy human cells with reduced MHC I

Natural Killer Cells

- CD16 on surface
  - Binds Fc of IgG → enhanced activity
  - Antibody-dependent cell-mediated cytotoxicity
- CD56
  - Also called NCAM (Neural Cell Adhesion Molecule)
  - Expressed on surface of NK cells (useful marker)
  - Also found in brain and neuromuscular junctions
  - Aids in binding to other cells

ADCC
Antibody-dependent cellular cytotoxicity

- Antibodies coat pathogen or cell
- Pathogen destroyed by immune cells
- Non-phagocytic process
- Classic examples: NK cells and Eosinophils

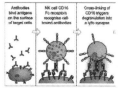

Satchmo2000/Wikipedia

ADCC
Antibody-dependent cellular cytotoxicity

- Natural Killer Cells
  - IgG binds to pathogen-infected cells
  - CD16 on NK binds Fc of IgG
  - NKC kills cell
- Eosinophils
  - IgE binds to pathogens, especially large parasites
  - Eosinophils bind Fc of IgE
  - Release of toxic enzymes onto parasite

Natural Killer Cells

- Lymphocytes (same lineage as T-cells and B-cells)
- Do not mature in thymus
- No memory
- Do not require antigen presentation by MHC

Eosinophils, Mast Cells, Basophils

- All contain granules with destructive enzymes
- All can be activated/triggered by IgE antibodies
- Important for defense against parasites (helminths)
  - Too large for phagocytosis
- Release of toxic substances kills parasite
- Main medical relevance is in allergic disease

Thymus

- Cortex:
  - Positive selection
  - Thymus epithelial cells express MHC
  - T-cells tested for binding to self MHC complexes
  - Weak binding: apoptosis
- Medulla
  - Negative selection
  - Thymus epithelial cells and dendritic cells express self antigens
  - T-cells tested for binding to self antigens and MHC
  - Excessive binding: apoptosis

Public Domain/Wikipedia

Thymus

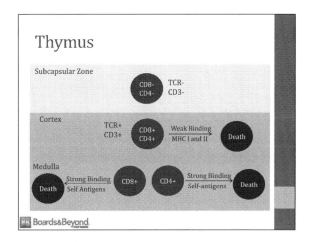

AIRE Genes

- Autoimmune regulator (AIRE)
- Genes responsible for expression self antigens
- Mutations → autoimmune disease
- Clinical consequences:
  - Recurrent candida infections
  - Chronic mucocutaneous candidiasis
  - Hypoparathyroidism
  - Adrenal insufficiency

B-cells

B-cells

Jason Ryan, MD, MPH

B cells

- Part of adaptive immune system
- Lymphocytes (T-cells, NK cells)
- Millions of B cells in human body
- Each recognizes a unique antigen
- Once recognizes antigen: synthesizes antibodies
- Antibodies attach to pathogens → elimination

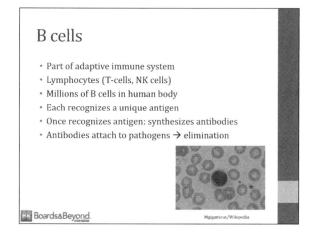

Mgiganteus/Wikipedia

B cell Receptor

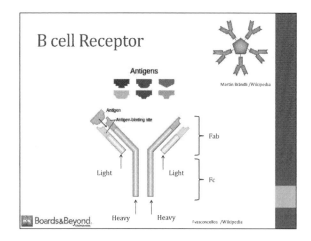

Martin Brändli /Wikipedia

F.vasconcellos /Wikipedia

B Cell Receptor

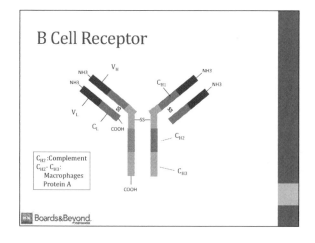

B cell Diversity

- Millions of B cells with unique antigen receptors
- More unique receptors than genes
- If one gene = one receptor, how can this be?
- Answer: Rearrangements of genetic building blocks

B Cell Receptor

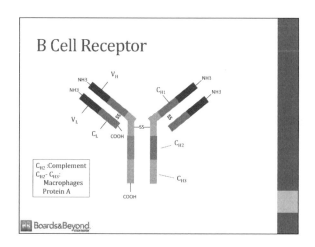

VDJ Rearrangement
Heavy Chain

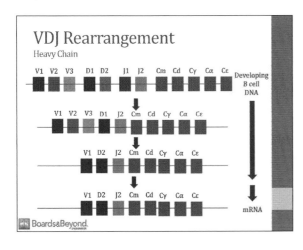

VDJ Rearrangement

- Heavy chain
  - V (~50 genes), D (~25 genes), J (~6 genes)
  - Chromosome 14
- Light chain
  - V/J gene rearrangements
- Random combination heavy + light = more diversity
- Key point: Small number genes = millions receptors

B cell Activation

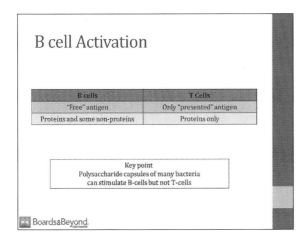

B cells	T Cells
"Free" antigen	Only "presented" antigen
Proteins and some non-proteins	Proteins only

Key point
Polysaccharide capsules of many bacteria
can stimulate B-cells but not T-cells

B cell Activation

- Two types of activation
  - T-cell dependent (proteins)
  - T-cell independent (non-proteins)
- For T-cell dependent, two signals required:
  - #1: Crosslinking of receptors bound to antigen
  - #2: T cell binding (T-cell dependent activation)

Receptor Crosslinking

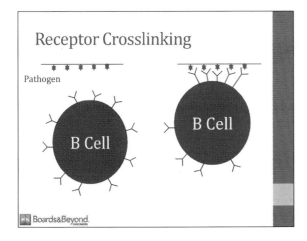

Pathogen

T Cell Dependent Activation

- B cell can present antigen to T-cells via MHC Class II
  - Binds MHC Class II to T cell receptor
- Other T-cell to B-cell interactions also occur
- CD40 (B cells) to CD40 ligand (T cell)
  - Required for class switching
- B7 (B cells) to CD28 (T cell)
  - Required for stimulation of T-cell cytokine production

T Cell Dependent Activation

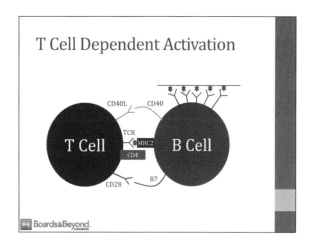

T Cell Dependent Activation

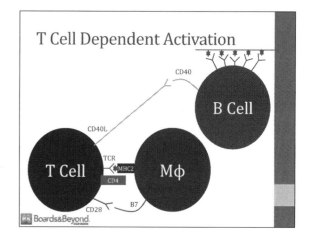

T Cell Independent Activation

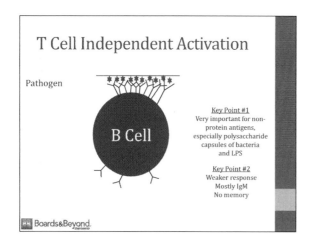

Pathogen

Key Point #1
Very important for non-protein antigens, especially polysaccharide capsules of bacteria and LPS

Key Point #2
Weaker response
Mostly IgM
No memory

B Cell Activation

T Cell Dependent	T Cell Independent
Protein antigens only	Non-protein
Vigorous response	Relatively weak response
Class switching (IgG, IgA, IgE)	Mostly IgM
Memory	No-memory

Important for polysaccharide capsules of bacteria and LPS

Conjugated Vaccines

- Polysaccharide antigen
  - No T-cell stimulation
  - Poor B cell memory
  - Weak immune response → weak protection
- Conjugated to peptide antigen
  - B-cells generate antibodies to polysaccharide
  - Protein antigen presented to T-cells
  - T-cells boost B-cell response
  - Strong immune response → strong protection

Conjugated Vaccines

- H. Influenza type B (Hib)
- Neisseria meningitidis
- Streptococcus pneumoniae

B Cell Surface Proteins

- Proteins for binding with T cells
  - CD40 (binding with T-cell CD40L)
  - MHC Class II
  - B7 (binds with CD28 on T cells)
- Other surface markers
  - CD19: All B cells
  - CD20: Most B cells, not plasma cells
  - CD21 (Complement, EBV)

Antibody Classes

Antibody class determined by Fc portion

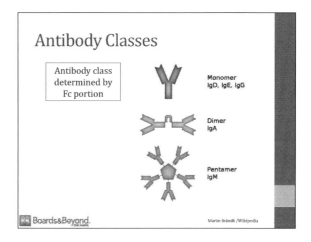

Monomer
IgD, IgE, IgG

Dimer
IgA

Pentamer
IgM

Martin Brändli /Wikipedia

Antibody Functions

- #1: Opsonization
  - Mark pathogens for phagocytosis
- #2: Neutralization
  - Block adherence to structures
- #3: Activate complement
  - "Classical" pathway activated by antibodies

Protein A

- Key virulence factor of Staph Aureus
- Part of peptidoglycan cell wall
- Binds Fc portion of IgG antibodies
- Prevents Mφ opsonization phagocytosis
- Prevents complement activation

Class Switching

- Activated B cells initially produce IgM
  - Can also produce small amount IgD
  - Significance of IgD not clear
- As B cell matures/proliferates, it can **switch class**
- Gene rearrangements produces IgG, IgA, IgE
- NOTE: No change in antibody specificity
- Triggers for class switching:
  - Cytokines (IL-4, IL-5 in Th2 response)
  - T-cell binding (CD40-CD40L)

VDJ Rearrangement
Heavy Chain

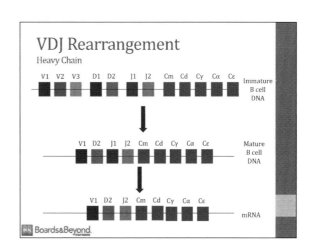

IgM

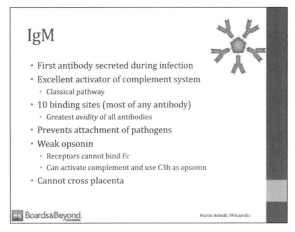

- First antibody secreted during infection
- Excellent activator of complement system
  - Classical pathway
- 10 binding sites (most of any antibody)
  - Greatest *avidity* of all antibodies
- Prevents attachment of pathogens
- Weak opsonin
  - Receptors cannot bind Fc
  - Can activate complement and use C3b as opsonin
- Cannot cross placenta

IgG

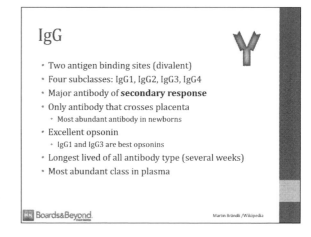

- Two antigen binding sites (divalent)
- Four subclasses: IgG1, IgG2, IgG3, IgG4
- Major antibody of **secondary response**
- Only antibody that crosses placenta
  - Most abundant antibody in newborns
- Excellent opsonin
  - IgG1 and IgG3 are best opsonins
- Longest lived of all antibody type (several weeks)
- Most abundant class in plasma

IgG

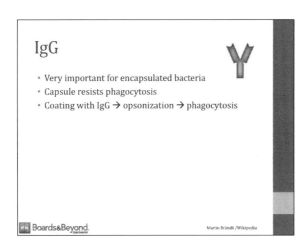

- Very important for encapsulated bacteria
- Capsule resists phagocytosis
- Coating with IgG → opsonization → phagocytosis

IgA

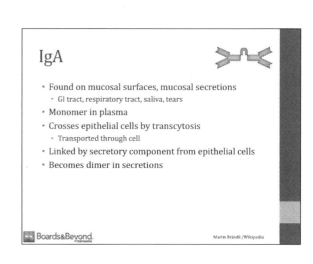

- Found on mucosal surfaces, mucosal secretions
  - GI tract, respiratory tract, saliva, tears
- Monomer in plasma
- Crosses epithelial cells by transcytosis
  - Transported through cell
- Linked by secretory component from epithelial cells
- Becomes dimer in secretions

IgA

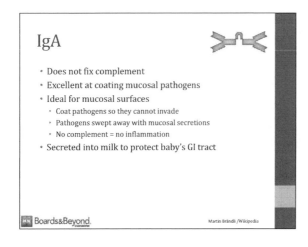

- Does not fix complement
- Excellent at coating mucosal pathogens
- Ideal for mucosal surfaces
  - Coat pathogens so they cannot invade
  - Pathogens swept away with mucosal secretions
  - No complement = no inflammation
- Secreted into milk to protect baby's GI tract

IgA

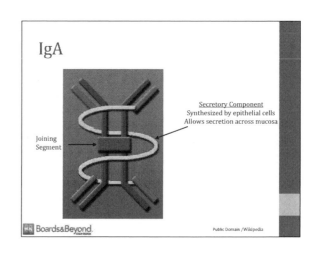

Secretory Component
Synthesized by epithelial cells
Allows secretion across mucosa

Joining Segment

Complement System

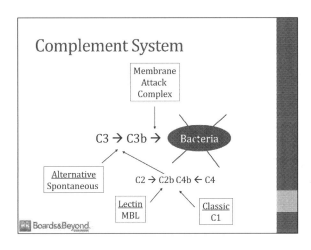

Membrane Attack Complex

- Stable C3b leads to formation of the MAC
- MAC formed from C5, C6, C7, C8, C9

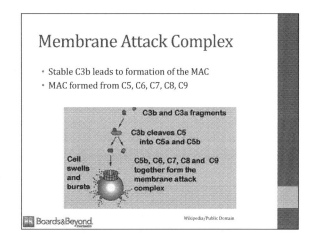

C5a

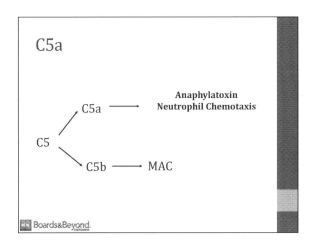

Complement System

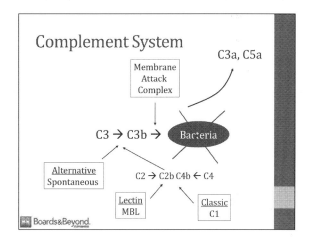

Inhibition of Complement

- Membrane proteins protect human cells
  - Decay Accelerating Factor (DAF/CD55)
  - MAC inhibitory protein (CD59)
- DAF disrupts C3b attachment
- CD59 disrupts MAC
- Especially important for protecting RBCs
- Deficiency of DAF or CD59 leads to hemolysis

PNH
Paroxysmal Nocturnal Hemoglobinuria

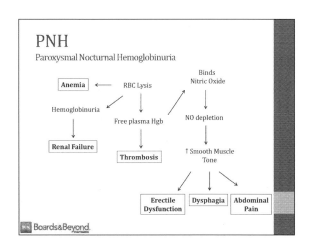

PNH
Paroxysmal Nocturnal Hemoglobinuria

- Classically causes sudden hemolysis at night
- Fatigue, dyspnea (anemia)
- Abdominal pain (smooth muscle tension)
- Thrombosis
  - Leading cause of death
  - Usually venous clots
  - Unusual locations: portal, mesenteric, cerebral veins

Inherited C3 Deficiency

- Recurrent infections encapsulated bacteria
  - Pneumococcal and H. flu pneumonia
  - Begins in infancy
- Immune complex (IC) deposition
  - IC cleared when they bind complement
  - Macrophages have complement receptors
  - C3 deficiency: glomerulonephritis from IC deposition
  - Other **type III hypersensitivity syndromes** can occur

C5-C9 Deficiency
Terminal complement pathway deficiency

- Like C3, impaired defense against encapsulated bugs
- Still have C3a (anaphylatoxin)
- Also have C3b (opsonin for macrophages)
- Recurrent Neisseria infections
- Most often meningitis

Hereditary Angioedema

- Deficiency of C1 inhibitor protein
- Many functions beyond complement system
- Breaks down bradykinin (vasodilator)
- Deficiency leads to high bradykinin levels
- Episodes of swelling/edema

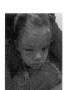

Hereditary Angioedema

- Recurrent episodes swelling without urticaria
- Begins in childhood
- Swelling of skin, GI tract, upper airway
- Airway swelling can be fatal
- Diagnosis: Low C4 level
  - Lack of C1 inhibitor
  - Consumption of C4
- Can treat with C1 inhibitor concentrate

ACE Inhibitors

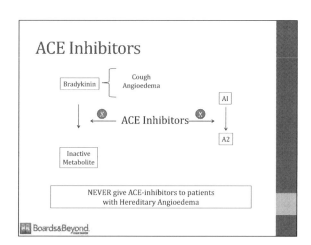

NEVER give ACE-inhibitors to patients with Hereditary Angioedema

C3 Nephritic Factor

- Autoantibody
- Stabilizes C3 convertase
- Overactivity of classical pathway
- Found in >80% patients with MPGN II
- Leads to inflammation, hypocomplementemia

Hypocomplementemia

- CH50
  - Patient serum added to sheep RBCs with antibodies
  - Tests classical pathway
  - Need all complement factors (C1-C9) for normal result
  - Normal range: 150 to 250 units/mL
- C3 or C4 level
  - Low in many complement mediated diseases (consumption)
  - Lupus and lupus nephritis
  - MPGN
  - Post-streptococcal glomerulonephritis

Lymph Nodes and Spleen

Jason Ryan, MD, MPH

Boards&Beyond

Lymph

- Interstitial fluid from tissues
- Drains into lymphatic system
- Circulates through lymph nodes
- Eventually drains into subclavian veins

Boards&Beyond

Lymphoid Organs

- Primary lymphoid organs
  - Sites of lymphocyte formation
  - Bone marrow, Thymus
  - Create B and T cells
- Secondary lymphoid organs
  - B cells and T cells proliferate
  - Lymph nodes
  - Spleen
  - Peyer's patches
  - Tonsils

Boards&Beyond

Lymph Nodes

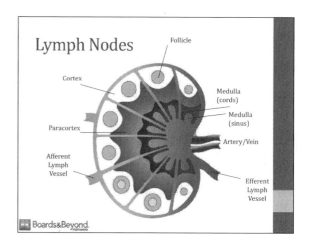

Boards&Beyond

Lymph Nodes

- Lymph fluid drains from site of infection
  - Dendritic cells activated
  - Express MHC I, MHC II, B7
  - Enter lymph carrying processed antigens
  - Free antigens also carried with lymph
- Lymph enters nodes
  - Many B and T cells waiting for matching antigen
- Dendritic cells present to T cells
- APCs in lymph nodes to process antigen
- B cells react to antigen
- Result: Generation of adaptive immune response

Boards&Beyond

Lymphoid Follicles

- Found in cortex of lymph nodes
- Site of B-cell activation
- Contain follicular dendritic cells
  - Different from tissue dendritic cells
  - Permanent cells of lymph nodes
  - Surface receptors bind complement-antigen complexes
  - Allows easy crosslinking of B cell receptors
- Special note: FDCs important reservoir for HIV
  - Early after infection large amounts HIV particles in FDCs

Boards&Beyond

Lymphoid Follicles

- Primary follicles
  - Inactive follicles
  - Follicular dendritic cells and B cells
- Secondary follicles
  - "Germinal center"
  - B cell growth and differentiation, class switching
  - Nearby helper T cells can bind → more growth

Lymphoid Follicles

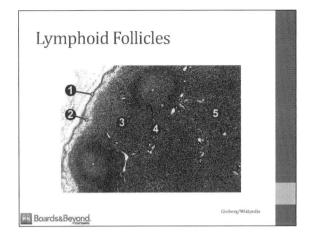

Gleiberg/Wikipedia

Paracortex

- Two key features:
  - #1: Contain T cells activated by dendritic cells and antigen
  - #2: Contain high endothelial venules
    - Vessels that allow B/T cell entry into node
- Engorged in immune response (swollen nodes)
- Underdeveloped in rare T-cell deficiency disorders
  - DiGeorge syndrome

Medulla

- Medullary sinuses (cavities)
  - Contain macrophages
  - Filters lymph → phagocytosis
- Medullary chords (tissue between cavities)
  - Contain plasma cells secreting antibodies

Spleen

- Filters blood (no lymph)
- All blood elements can enter
  - No high endothelial venules
  - No selective entry T and B cells

Wikipedia/Public Domain

Spleen

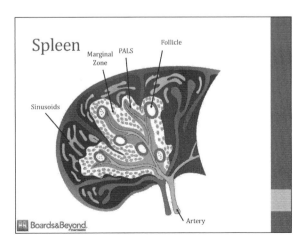

Spleen

- White pulp
  - Exposure to B and T cells
  - Exposure to macrophages
- Red pulp
  - Filters blood in sinusoids
  - Removes old RBCs (red)
  - Stores many platelets

White Pulp

- Marginal zone
  - Macrophages
  - Remove debris
  - Dendritic cells process antigen
- Follicles
  - B cells
- Periarteriolar lymphocyte sheath (PALS)
  - T cells

Sinusoids of Spleen

- Red pulp lined by vascular "sinusoids"
- Open endothelium → cells pass in/out
- Capillaries → cords → sinusoids
- Cords contain macrophages (filtration)

Splenic Dysfunction

- Increased risk from **encapsulated organisms**
- Loss of marginal zone macrophages → ↓ phagocytosis
- Also loss of opsonization:
  - ↓ IgM and IgG against capsules (splenic B cells)
  - Loss of IgG opsonization
  - ↓ complement against encapsulated bacteria
  - ↓ C3b opsonization

Splenic Dysfunction

- **Strep pneumo** is predominant pathogen for sepsis
  - Death in > 50% of patients
- Others: H. flu (Hib), Neisseria meningitidis
- Less common: Strep pyogenes, E coli, Salmonella
- Also malaria and babesia (RBC infections)

Ram e al; Infections of People with Complement Deficiencies and Patients Who Have Undergone Splenectomy Clin Microbiol Rev. 2010 Oct; 23(4): 740–780.

Splenic Dysfunction

- Splenectomy
  - Trauma
  - ITP (spleen site of phagocytosis of platelets)
  - Hereditary spherocytosis (minimizes anemia)
- Functional asplenia
  - Sickle cell anemia

Splenic Dysfunction

- Howell Jolly Bodies
  - Some RBCs leave marrow with nuclear remnants
  - Normally cleared by spleen
  - Presence in peripheral blood indicates splenic dysfunction
- Target cells
  - Also seen in liver disease, hemoglobin disorders
  - From too much surface area (membrane) or too little volume
  - Too much surface area: liver disease
  - Too little volume: hemoglobin disorders
- Thrombocytosis
  - Failure of spleen to remove platelets

Splenic Dysfunction

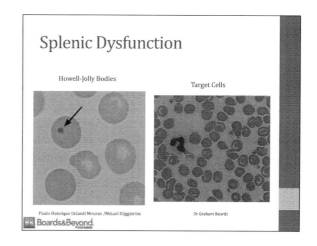

Howell-Jolly Bodies   Target Cells

Paulo Henrique Orlandi Mourao /Mikael Häggström   Dr Graham Beards

Hypersensitivity

Jason Ryan, MD, MPH

Boards&Beyond

Hypersensitivity

- Immune response that causes disease
- Exaggerated or inappropriate
- Allergic reactions = subtype of hypersensitivity

Boards&Beyond

Hypersensitivity

- First contact with antigen "sensitizes"
  - Generation of immune response
  - Antibodies, Memory cells
- Second contact → hypersensitivity
- Symptoms from overreaction of immune system
- Four patterns of underlying immune response
- Type I, II, III, IV

Boards&Beyond

Type I

- Immediate reaction to an antigen (minutes)
  - Pollen, pet dander, peanuts
- Pre-formed IgE antibodies (primary exposure)
- Antibodies bound to mast cells
- Antigen binds and cross links IgE
- Mast cell degranulation

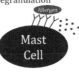

Boards&Beyond

Type I Immunology

- Susceptible individuals make IgE to antigens
- Majority of people make IgG
  - IgG does not trigger hypersensitivity response
- IgE results from:
  - B cell class switching
  - Driven by Th2 cells (humoral response)
  - **IL-4 is key cytokine** for IgE production
- No complement
  - IgE does not activate complement

Boards&Beyond

Type I Symptoms

- Skin: Urticaria (hives)
- Respiratory tract
  - Rhinitis
  - Wheezing (asthma)
- Eyes: Conjunctivitis
- GI tract: Diarrhea

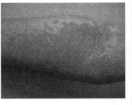

Boards&Beyond

James Heilman, MD/Wikipedia

Anaphylaxis

* Systemic type I hypersensitivity reaction
* Itching, diffuse hives/erythema
* Respiratory distress from bronchoconstriction
* Hoarseness (laryngeal swelling/edema)
* Vomiting, cramps, diarrhea
* Shock and death
* Treatment: Epinephrine

Boards&Beyond

Atopy

* Genetic predisposition to localized hypersensitivity
* Urticaria, rhinitis, asthma
* Usually positive family history of similar reaction

Boards&Beyond

Type I Examples

* Asthma
* Penicillin drug allergy
* Seasonal allergies (allergic rhinitis)
* Allergic conjunctivitis
* Peanut allergy (children)
* Shellfish (food allergy)

Boards&Beyond

Type I

* Early symptoms
    * Occur within minutes
    * Degranulation → release of pre-formed mediators (histamine)
    * Synthesis/release of leukotrienes, prostaglandins
    * Edema, redness, itching
* Late symptoms
    * ~6 hours later
    * Synthesis/release of cytokines
    * Influx of inflammatory cells (neutrophils, eosinophils)
    * Induration

Boards&Beyond

Type I Mediators

* Histamine
    * Vasodilation (warmth)
    * Increased permeability venules (swelling)
    * Smooth muscle contraction (bronchospasm)
* Leukotrienes, prostaglandins and thromboxanes
    * Derived from arachidonic acid

Boards&Beyond

Eicosanoids

Lipids (cell membranes)

↓ Phospholipase A2

Arachidonic acid

Lipoxygenase   Cyclooxygenase

Leukotrienes

Thromboxanes

Prostaglandins

Boards&Beyond

Eicosanoids
Type I Hypersensitivity

Mediator	Effects
PGE_2	Redness (vasodilation) Edema (permeability) Fever (hypothalamus) Pain (nerves)
PGD_2	Bronchoconstriction Eosinophil infiltration
LTC4/LTD4	Vasoconstriction Bronchoconstrictors
LTB4	Neutrophil, eosinophil chemotaxis

Ricciotti E, FitzGerald G; **Prostaglandins and Inflammation**
Arterioscler Thromb Vasc Biol. 2011 May; 31(5): 986–1000.

Boards&Beyond.

Other Type I Mediators

- ECF-A
  - Eosinophil chemotactic factor of anaphylaxis
  - Preformed in mast cells
  - Attracts eosinophils (various roles)
- Serotonin
  - Preformed in mast cells, causes vasodilation
- Platelet activating factor
  - Bronchoconstriction
- Neutral proteases (chymase, tryptase)
- Heparin (anticoagulant)

IgE, Mast Cells, Basophils, and Eosinophils. J Allergy Clin Immunol. 2010 Feb; 125(2 Suppl 2): S73–S80.

Boards&Beyond.

Testing and Desensitization

- Testing for IgE
  - Pinprick/puncture of skin
  - Intradermal injection
  - Positive response: wheal formation
- Desensitization
  - Gradual administration of increasing amounts of allergen
  - Response changes IgE → IgG
  - IgG antibodies can "block" mediator release
  - "Modified Th2 response"

Boards&Beyond.

Type II

- Antibodies (IgG/IgM) directed against tissue antigens
- Binding to normal structures
- Three mechanisms of tissue/cell damage
  - Phagocytosis
  - Complement-mediated lysis
  - Antibody-dependent cytotoxicity

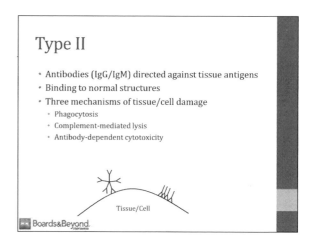

Tissue/Cell

Boards&Beyond.

Type II

- Phagocytosis
  - Fc receptors or C3b receptors on phagocytes
- Complement
  - IgM or IgG → classical complement cascade
  - Formation of MAC → cell death
- ADCC
  - Antibody-dependent cell-mediated cytotoxicity
  - Natural killer cells bind Fc portion IgG

Boards&Beyond.

Type II Examples

- Rheumatic fever
  - Strep antibodies cross-react with cardiac myocytes
- Exposure to wrong blood type
  - RBC lysis by circulating IgG
  - Erythroblastosis fetalis
- Autoimmune hemolytic anemia
  - Methyldopa and penicillin: drugs bind to surface of RBCs
  - Mycoplasma pneumonia: Induces RBC antibodies

Boards&Beyond.

Type II Examples

- Pemphigus vulgaris
  - Antibodies against desmosomes in epidermis
- Goodpasture syndrome
  - Nephritic syndrome and pulmonary hemorrhage
  - Type IV collagen antibodies
- Myasthenia gravis
  - Antibodies against Ach receptors

Type III

- Antigen-antibody (IgG) complexes form
- Activate complement → tissue/cell damage
- Generalized: Serum sickness
- Localized: Arthus reaction

Martin Brändli /Wikipedia

Generalized Type III
Serum sickness

- IC in plasma → systemic disease
  - Usually IgG or IgM (complement activators)
- Deposit in various tissues
  - Skin
  - Kidneys
  - Joints
- Trigger immune response
  - Complement activation
  - Activation of macrophages and neutrophils (Fc receptors)

Generalized Type III
Serum sickness

- Historical description:
  - Horse plasma used for passive immunization
  - ~5-10 days later triad: **Fever, rash, arthralgias**
- Antibodies to horse serum antigens
- IC deposits in skin, joints

Generalized Type III
Serum sickness

- Urticaria or palpable purpura
- Low serum complement levels
- Elevated sedimentation rate
- Diffuse lymphadenopathy
- Acute glomerulonephritis

Generalized Type III
Serum sickness

- Classic serum sickness
  - Rabies or tetanus anti-toxin
  - Rarely penicillin: drug acts as a "hapten"
  - Monoclonal antibodies (rituximab, infliximab)
- Other Type III diseases
  - Post-strep glomerulonephritis
  - Systemic lupus erythematosus (Anti-DNA antibodies)
  - Polyarteritis nodosa (Hep B antigens)

Localized Type III
Arthus Reaction

* Local tissue reaction, usually in the skin
* Injection of antigen
* Preformed antibodies in plasma/tissue
* Formation of immune complexes

Localized Type III
Arthus Reaction

* Local immune complexes form
  * 4-10 hours after injection
  * Contrast with Type I reaction in minutes
  * Complement activation, edema, necrosis
* Immunofluorescent staining
  * Antibodies, complement in vessel walls

Localized Type III
Arthus Reaction

* Reported with skin injections:
  * Tetanus, diphtheria, hep B vaccines
  * Insulin
  * Swelling, redness at site hours after injection
* Hypersensitivity pneumonitis
  * Farmer's lung
  * Hypersensitivity reaction to environmental antigen

Type IV
Delayed-type hypersensitivity

* Cell-mediated reaction
* No antibodies (different from I, II, III)
* Memory T-cells initiate immune response

Type IV
Delayed-type hypersensitivity

* Classic example: PPD test (tuberculosis)
  * Tuberculin protein injected into skin
  * Previously exposed person has memory T-cells
  * CD4 T-cells recognize protein on APCs (MHC II)
  * Th1 response
  * IFN-γ activates macrophages
  * IL-12 from macrophages stimulates Th1 cells
  * Result: Redness, induration 24 to 72 hours later

Type IV Examples

* Immune response to many pathogens:
  * Mycobacteria
  * Fungi
* Contact dermatitis (i.e. poison ivy)
  * Chemicals (oils) attach to skin cells
  * Involves CD8 T-cells that attack skin cells
  * Erythema, itching
  * 12 to 48hrs after exposure (contrast with type I)
* Multiple sclerosis
  * Myelin basic protein

Transplants

Transplants

Jason Ryan, MD, MPH

Organ Transplants US 2014

Organ	Number
Kidney	17,000
Liver	6,700
Heart	2,600
Lung	1,900
Pancreas	250

Usually indicated when organ has failed

Bone Marrow Transplants

- About 17,000 per year in united states
- Abolish bone marrow with chemotherapy
- Reconstitute all cell lines with donor marrow
  - Sometimes autotransplant
  - Blood type can change!

Bone Marrow Transplants

- Malignancy (leukemia/lymphoma)
- Inherited red cell disorders
  - Pure red cell aplasia, sickle cell disease, beta-thalassemia
- Marrow failure (aplastic anemia, Fanconi anemia)
- Metabolic disorders
  - Adrenoleukodystrophy, Gaucher's disease
- Inherited immune disorders
  - Severe combined immunodeficiency, Wiskott-Aldrich

Transplant Vocabulary

Graft Type	Features
Autograft	Donor-recipient same person
Syngenetic Graft	Identical twins
Xenograft	Different species
Allograft	Same species

Matching

- Goal is to "match" transplanted tissue
  - Recipient and donor tissue same/similar
- Failure to match leads to rejection of transplant
  - Immune system attacks transplant as foreign

Features of a Good Match

* Same blood type
* Same (or close) MHC I and II molecules
* Negative cross-matching screen
  * Test of donor cells against recipient plasma
  * Screen for antibodies

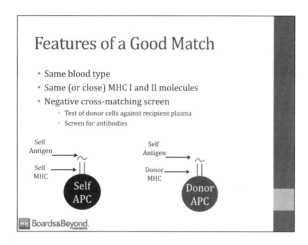

MHC Matching

* Donor cells express MHC I
  * If different from recipient, CD8 cells will react
* MHC Class II also expressed
  * Donor APCs may be carried along
  * Vascular endothelial cells may express MHC II

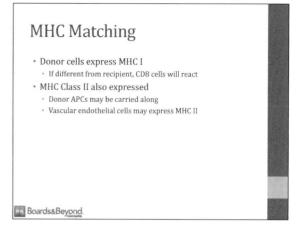

Human Leukocyte Antigens
HLAs

* Antigens that make up MHC class I and II molecules
* If different between donor-recipient, immune system will classify donor tissue as foreign

HLA Matching

* Genes on chromosome 6 determine "HLA type"
* MHC Class I
  * Genes: HLA-A, HLA-B, HLA-C
* MHC Class II
  * HLA-DR, -DM, -DO, -DP, -DQ
* Highly polymorphic
  * Many HLA antigens (i.e. more than 50 HLA-A)
  * Subtypes numbered: A1, A2, A3, etc.
* If donor-recipient do not match: rejection

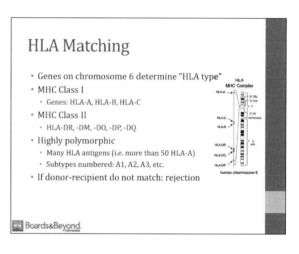

HLA Subtypes

* Some associated with **autoimmune** diseases
* Example: B27
  * Higher risk of ankylosing spondylitis
  * Also psoriasis, inflammatory bowel disease, Reiter's syndrome
* Example: A3
  * Higher risk of hemochromatosis

HLA Matching

* Two **sets** of HLA genes per patient
  * All HLAs transferred en bloc from each parent
  * 1 set from mother (i.e. A2, B3, etc.)
  * 1 set from father
* Sibling has 25% chance of perfect match

MHC Matching

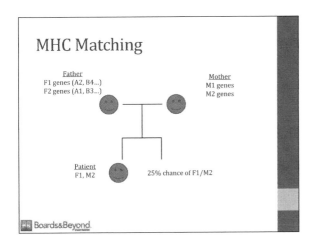

Father
F1 genes (A2, B4...)
F2 genes (A1, B3...)

Mother
M1 genes
M2 genes

Patient
F1, M2

25% chance of F1/M2

The "Perfect" Match

- Two-haplotype match
  - Still some degree of incompatibility
  - Minor histocompatibility antigens
- Identical twins
  - Only time when true "perfect" match exists

MHC Matching

- Most important HLA genes for solid organ transplants:
  - HLA-A, HLA-B, HLA-DR
  - Sometimes called a "6 out of 6 match"
- More genes sometimes tested
  - If HLA-C and HLA-DQ tests, "10 out of 10 match"

Source: American Society for Histocompatibility and Immunogenetics (ASHI)

Bone Marrow Transplants

- Chemotherapy to abolish recipient bone marrow
- Grafted cells must replenish all cell lines
- Matched for HLA-A, -B, -DR, also HLA-C
  - Sometimes also -DQ, -DP
- Two problems with mismatch:
  - Rejection of new cells
  - Graft versus host disease

Graft Versus Host Disease

- Mostly a complication of bone marrow transplant
- Donated (grafted) T-cells (CD8) react to recipient cells
  - See recipient cells as foreign
  - Opposite of rejection
- Symptoms GVHD
  - Skin: Rash
  - GI Tract: Diarrhea, abdominal pain
  - Liver: ↑LFTs, ↑bilirubin

Graft Versus Host Disease

- Small degree GVHD may be good
  - New WBCs kill residual cancer cells
  - Graft-vs-leukemia (GVL) effect
  - Associated with increased overall survival (less relapse)

Rejection

- Hyperacute (minutes)
- Acute (weeks-months)
- Chronic (years)

Hyperacute Rejection

- Within minutes of transplantation
- Caused by preformed antibodies in recipient
  - Against ABO or HLA antigens
  - Antibodies formed from previous exposure foreign antigens
  - Pregnancy, blood transfusion, previous transplantation
  - Prevented by cross-matching screen

MULLEY W, KANELLIS J. Understanding crossmatch testing in organ transplantation: A case-based guide for the general nephrologist. Nephrology 16 (2011) 125–133

Hyperacute Rejection

- Blood vessels spasm
- Intravascular coagulation
- Ischemia ("white rejection")
- Rare, usually not treatable

Acute Rejection

- Weeks/months after transplant
- Recipients T cells react to graft (via HLA)
- Cell-mediated immune response
- CD8 T-cells very important
- Biopsy: Infiltrates of **lymphocytes**/mononuclear cells
- Treatable with immunosuppression

Chronic Rejection

- Months or years after transplant
- Inflammation and **fibrosis**, especially vessels
  - Kidneys: fibrosis of capillaries, glomeruli
  - Heart: Narrowing coronary arteries
  - Lungs: bronchiolitis obliterans
- Complex, incompletely understood process
- Involves cell-mediated and humoral systems

Immune Deficiency Syndromes

Jason Ryan, MD, MPH

Boards&Beyond

Immune Deficiency
General Principles

- Loss of T-cells, B-cells, Granulocytes, Complement
- Acquired: HIV, Chemotherapy
- Genetic/Congenital:
  - Usually presents in infancy with recurrent infections

Boards&Beyond

X-linked Agammaglobulinemia
Bruton's Agammaglobulinemia

- X-linked
- Failure of B cell precursors to become B cells
- Light chains not produced
- Defect in Bruton tyrosine kinase (BTK) gene
- Symptoms begin ~6 months of age
  - Loss of maternal antibodies

Boards&Beyond

X-linked Agammaglobulinemia
Bruton's Agammaglobulinemia

- Recurrent respiratory bacterial infections
  - Loss of opsonization by antibodies
  - H. Flu, Strep pneumo are common
  - Classic presentation: Recurrent otitis media +/- sinusitis/PNA
- GI pathogen infections (loss of IgA)
  - Enteroviruses (echo, polio, coxsackie)
  - Giardia (GI parasite)

Boards&Beyond

X-linked Agammaglobulinemia
Bruton's Agammaglobulinemia

- Key findings:
  - Mature B cells (CD19, CD20, BCR) absent in peripheral blood
  - Underdeveloped germinal centers of lymph nodes
  - Absence of antibodies (all classes)
- Treatment: IVIG

Boards&Beyond

Selective IgA Deficiency

- Very common syndrome in US (~1 in 600)
- Defective IgA B-cells (exact mechanism unknown)
- Most patients asymptomatic
- Symptomatic patients:
  - Recurrent sinus, pulmonary infections
  - Otitis media, sinusitis, pneumonia
  - Recurrent diarrheal illnesses from Giardiasis
- Blood transfusions → anaphylaxis
  - IgA in blood products
  - Antibodies against IgA in IgA deficient patients
- SLE and RA are common (20-30%)

Boards&Beyond

Selective IgA Deficiency

- Diagnosis:
  - Serum IgA < 7mg/dl
  - Normal IgG, IgM
- Treatment:
  - Prophylactic antibiotics
  - IVIG
- Special features: False positive β-HCG test
  - Heterophile antibodies produced in IgA deficiency
  - Lead to false positive β-HCG
  - Up to 30% IgA deficient patients test positive for β-HCG

CVID
Common Variable Immunodeficiency

- Defective B cell maturation
- Loss of plasma cells and antibodies
- Many underlying genetic causes
  - Most cases due to unknown cause
  - 10+ genes mutations associated with CVID
  - Often sporadic – no family history
- Normal B cell count, absence of antibodies
  - Usually IgG
  - Sometimes IgA and IgM (variable)

CVID
Common Variable Immunodeficiency

- Similar to X-linked Agammaglobulinemia
  - Recurrent respiratory bacterial infections
  - Enteroviruses, Giardiasis
- Key differences:
  - Not X-linked (affects females)
  - Later onset (majority 20-45 years old)
- ↑ frequency other diseases:
  - RA, pernicious anemia, lymphoma

B Cell Disorders

	IgA Def	Bruton's	CVID
B Cells	Normal	↓	Normal
Antibodies	↓ IgA	↓ IgA, IgM, IgG	↓ IgA, IgM, IgG
Symptoms	Sinopulmonary GI	Sinopulmonary GI	Sinopulmonary GI
Special Features	False + β-HCG SLE/RA	Infancy	20s-40s Autoimmune Lymphoma

Thymic Aplasia
DiGeorge Syndrome

- Failure of 3rd/4th pharyngeal pouch to form

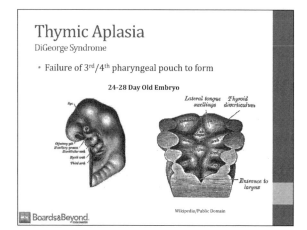

24-28 Day Old Embryo

Wikipedia/Public Domain

Thymic Aplasia
DiGeorge Syndrome

- Most cases: 22q11 chromosomal deletion
  - Key point: Not familial
- Classic triad:
  - Loss of thymus (Loss of T-cells, recurrent infections)
  - Loss of parathyroid glands (hypocalcemia, tetany)
  - Congenital heart defects ("conotruncal")
- Heart Defects:
  - Abnormal aortic arch
  - Truncus arteriosus
  - Tetralogy of Fallot
  - ASDs/VSDs

Thymic Aplasia
DiGeorge Syndrome

- Immune symptoms
  - Recurrent infections
  - Viral, fungal, protozoal, intracellular bacteria
  - Immune symptoms sometimes improve
- Cleft palate, mandible problems also common

Thymic Aplasia
Key Findings

- No thymus shadow on CXR
  - Thymus large in newborns
  - Faint white shadow on chest x-ray
  - Also seen in SCID (without ↓Ca, facial/heart abnormalities)
- Low T-cell count
- Underdeveloped T-cell structures
  - Paracortex in lymph nodes
  - Peri-arteriolar sheaths in spleen
- Treatment:
  - Thymic transplantation
  - Hematopoietic cell transplantation

Hyper-IgE Syndrome
Job's Syndrome

- Rare syndrome, poorly understood
- Immune symptoms with skin/bone findings
- Defective CD4+ **Th17 cells**
  - Failure to produce IL-17
- **Loss of attraction of neutrophils**
- Defects of STAT3 signaling pathway
  - Signal transducer and activator of transcription
  - Activated by cytokines
- Overproduction IgE, loss of IFN-γ
- Characteristic labs: ↑IgE, ↓IFN-γ

Hyper-IgE Syndrome
Job's Syndrome

- Skin findings
  - First few weeks of life
  - Diffuse eczema (also crusted lesions, boils, etc.)
  - Histamine release → itching
- Staph abscesses face, scalp
  - Classically "**cold**" - lacking warmth/redness of inflammation
  - Loss of cytokine production
- Recurrent sinusitis, otitis (often without fever)
- Facial deformities (broad nasal bridge)
- Retained primary teeth (two rows of teeth!)

Wikipedia/Public Domain

Hyper-IgE Syndrome
Job's Syndrome

- Classic case:
  - Newborn baby
  - Deformed face/teeth
  - Diffuse rash
  - **Skin abscesses that are "cold"**
  - Recurrent infections without fever
  - Labs: Elevated IgE

Chronic mucocutaneous candidiasis

- Defect in autoimmune regulator (AIRE) genes
- AIRE Function #1:
  - Associates with Dectin-1 receptor
  - Dectin-1 responds to Candida antigens
  - Result of defect: Recurrent candida infections
- AIRE Function #2:
  - Promotes self antigens production in thymus
  - Self antigens presented to T-cells (negative selection)
  - Result of defect: Autoimmune T-cells
  - Endocrine dysfunction (parathyroid/adrenal)

Chronic mucocutaneous candidiasis

- T-cell dysfunction (cell-mediated defect)
  - Th1 cytokines: ↓IL-2, ↓IFN-γ
  - ↑IL-10 (anti-inflammatory cytokine)
  - NOT due to antibody or B-cell deficiencies
- T cells fail to react to candida antigens

D Lilic. New perspectives on the immunology of chronic mucocutaneous candidiasis. Curr Opin Infect Dis. 2002; 15(2):143-7

Boards&Beyond

Chronic mucocutaneous candidiasis

- Chronic skin, mucous membrane candida infections
  - Thrush
  - Skin
  - Esophagus
- Associated with **endocrine dysfunction**:
  - Hypoparathyroidism
  - Adrenal failure
- Classic case:
  - Child with recurrent thrush, diaper rash

Boards&Beyond

Candida Infections

- T-cells important for mucosal defense
  - Example: HIV patients often get thrush (↓CD4)
- Neutrophils important for systemic defense
  - HIV patients rarely get candidemia
  - No candidemia in CMC
  - Chemo patients at risk for candidemia (neutropenia)

Boards&Beyond

SCID
Severe Combined Immunodeficiency

- Loss of cell-mediated and humoral immunity
  - Usually primary T cell problem
  - Loss of B-cells, antibodies usually secondary

Boards&Beyond

SCID
Severe Combined Immunodeficiency

- T-cell/B cell areas absent/diminished:
  - Loss of thymic shadow
  - Loss of germinal centers in nodes
- Susceptible to many infections
  - Thrush, bacterial, viral, fungal
  - Babies: Thrush, diaper rash, failure to thrive
- Death unless bone marrow transplant

Boards&Beyond

SCID
Severe Combined Immunodeficiency

- Most common forms are X-linked (boys)
  - Mutation of γ subunit of cytokine receptors
  - Gene: IL2RG (interleukin-2 receptor gamma gene)
- Also caused by adenosine deaminase gene deficiency
- Newborn screening:
  - Maternal T-cells may falsely indicate normal counts
  - TRECs (T-cell receptor excision circles)
  - Circular DNA formed in normal T-cells in the thymus
  - Mandated in many states

Boards&Beyond

SCID
Severe Combined Immunodeficiency

- Classic case:
  - Infant with recurrent infections
  - Multiple systems: otitis, GI, candida (skin)
  - Absent thymic shadow
  - Normal calcium/heart (contrast with DiGeorge)

ADA
Adenosine Deaminase Deficiency

- Excess dATP
- Believed to inhibit ribonucleotide reductase
  - Ribonucleotides synthesized first (A, G, C, U)
  - Converted to deoxyribonucleotides by RR
- Result: ↓ DNA synthesis → B/T cell dysfunction

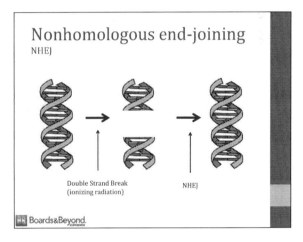

Ataxia Telangiectasia

- Autosomal recessive genetic disorder
- Defective ATM gene on chromosome 11
  - Ataxia Telangiectasia Mutated gene
  - Repairs double stranded DNA breaks
  - Nonhomologous end-joining (NHEJ)
  - Result: Failure to repair DNA mutations
- Hypersensitivity of DNA to ionizing radiation

Nonhomologous end-joining
NHEJ

Double Strand Break
(ionizing radiation)   NHEJ

Ataxia Telangiectasia

- Mix of systems involved with varying findings
  - CNS (ataxia)
  - Skin (telangiectasias)
  - Immune system (infections, malignancies)
- Presents in childhood with progressive symptoms
- Usually begins with gait and balance problems

Ataxia Telangiectasia

- Cerebellar atrophy
  - Ataxia in 1st year of life
- Telangiectasias
  - Dilation of capillary vessels on skin
- Repeated sinus/respiratory infections
  - Low levels immunoglobulins, especially IgA and IgG
- High risk of cancer (lymphomas)
- Commonly identified lab abnormalities:
  - Most consistent lab finding: ↑AFP
  - Low IgA level

Hyper-IgM Syndrome

- Class switching disorder
  - Failure of B cells (CD40) to T cell (CD40L) binding
  - 70% cases: Defective CD40L gene (**T-cell problem**)
- B cells make IgM only
- Labs show ↑IgM, all other antibodies absent
- Most common form X-linked (boys)

T Cell Dependent Activation

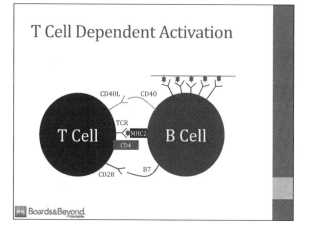

Hyper-IgM Syndrome

- Recurrent bacterial infections in infancy
  - Sinus and pulmonary infections
  - Pneumonia, sinusitis, otitis media
  - Mostly caused by encapsulated bacteria (S. pneumo, H. flu)
- Also opportunistic infections
  - Pneumocystis, Cryptosporidium, Histoplasmosis
- Loss of IgG opsonization

Wiskott-Aldrich Syndrome

- X linked disorder of WAS gene (WAS protein)
- WASp absence/dysfunction
  - Necessary for T-cell **cytoskeleton** maintenance
  - This forms "immunologic synapse"
  - T-cells cannot properly react to APCs
- Can worsen with age
- Immune dysfunction, ↓platelets, eczema
- Elevated IgE and IgA common (eczema)
- Treatment: Bone marrow transplant

Wiskott-Aldrich Syndrome

- Classic case
  - Male infant
  - 6 months old (maternal antibodies fade)
  - Eczema
  - Bleeding, petechiae (low platelets)
  - Recurrent infections

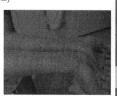

Wikipedia/Public Domain

Leukocyte Adhesion Deficiency

- Defective neutrophil/lymphocyte migration
- Most common type: Type 1
  - Autosomal recessive defect in CD18
  - Also called Lymphocyte function associated antigen-1 (LFA1)
  - Forms beta subunit of several **integrins** (adhesion molecules)
  - WBCs (especially PMNs) cannot roll, migrate

Leukocyte Adhesion Deficiency

- Delayed separation of the umbilical cord
  - After cord cutting, inflammation occurs
  - Cord stump normally falls off 2-3 days
  - Delayed in LAD (sometimes 30+ days)
  - Classic presenting infection: omphalitis (stump infection)
- Other findings:
  - Recurrent bacterial infections
  - Elevated WBCs (neutrophilia) – especially during infections

Chediak-Higashi Syndrome

- Failure of lysosomes to fuse with phagosomes
- Mutation: lysosomal trafficking regulator (LYST) gene
  - Causes **microtubule** dysfunction
- Recurrent bacterial infections
  - Especially Staph and Strep
- Oculocutaneous albinism
  - Fair skin, blond hair, light blue eyes
- Children who survive → severe neuro impairment
  - Peripheral neuropathy: weakness and sensory deficits
  - Often wheelchair bound

CGD
Chronic Granulomatous Disease

- Loss of function of NADPH oxidase
- Phagocytes use NADPH oxidase to generate H_2O_2 from oxygen (respiratory burst)
- Catalase (-) bacteria generate their own H_2O_2 which phagocytes use despite enzyme deficiency
- Catalase (+) bacteria breakdown H_2O_2
  - Host cells have no H_2O_2 to use → recurrent infections
- Five organisms cause almost all CGD infections:
  - Staph aureus, Pseudomonas, Serratia, Nocardia, Aspergillus

Source: UpToDate

CGD
Chronic Granulomatous Disease

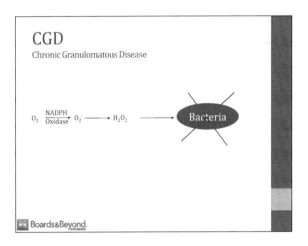

CGD
Chronic Granulomatous Disease

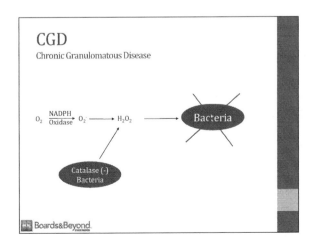

CGD
Chronic Granulomatous Disease

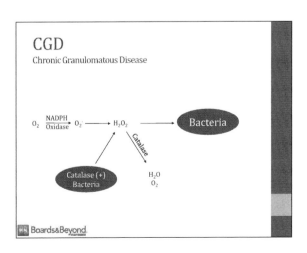

CGD

Chronic Granulomatous Disease

- Nitroblue tetrazolium test
  - Dye added to sample of neutrophils
  - Absence of NADPH oxidase → **cells do not turn blue**
  - A "negative" test indicates lack of enzyme
  - More blue, more NADPH oxidase present

Innate Immunity Defects

Disorder	Features
Leukocyte Adhesion Deficiency	↓↓ Neutrophil migration
Chediak-Higashi	Lysosome fusion; microtubules
Chronic Granulomatous Disease	↓↓ Respiratory Burst; Catalase (+) Infections

Glucocorticoids and NSAIDs

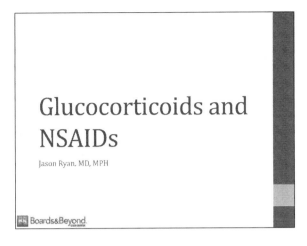

Glucocorticoids and NSAIDs

Jason Ryan, MD, MPH

Boards&Beyond

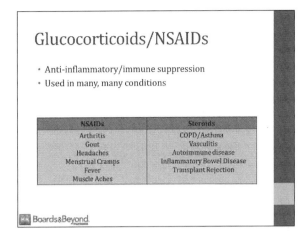

Glucocorticoids/NSAIDs

- Anti-inflammatory/immune suppression
- Used in many, many conditions

NSAIDs	Steroids
Arthritis	COPD/Asthma
Gout	Vasculitis
Headaches	Autoimmune disease
Menstrual Cramps	Inflammatory Bowel Disease
Fever	Transplant Rejection
Muscle Aches	

Boards&Beyond

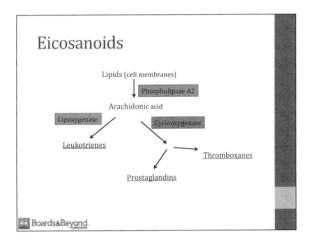

Eicosanoids

Lipids (cell membranes)

Phospholipase A2

Arachidonic acid

Lipoxygenase   Cyclooxygenase

Leukotrienes

Thromboxanes

Prostaglandins

Boards&Beyond

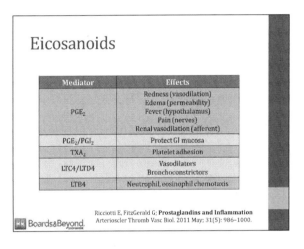

Eicosanoids

Mediator	Effects
PGE_2	Redness (vasodilation) Edema (permeability) Fever (hypothalamus) Pain (nerves) Renal vasodilation (afferent)
PGE_2/PGI_2	Protect GI mucosa
TXA_2	Platelet adhesion
LTC4/LTD4	Vasodilators Bronchoconstrictors
LTB4	Neutrophil, eosinophil chemotaxis

Ricciotti E, FitzGerald G; **Prostaglandins and Inflammation**
Arterioscler Thromb Vasc Biol. 2011 May; 31(5): 986–1000.

Boards&Beyond

Cyclooxygenase (COX)

- Two isoforms
- COX-1
  - Constitutively expressed
  - Important for GI mucosal function
- COX-2
  - Inducible in inflammatory cells

Boards&Beyond

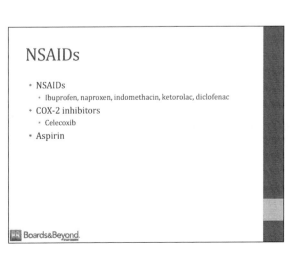

NSAIDs

- NSAIDs
  - Ibuprofen, naproxen, indomethacin, ketorolac, diclofenac
- COX-2 inhibitors
  - Celecoxib
- Aspirin

Boards&Beyond

NSAIDs

Ibuprofen, naproxen, indomethacin, ketorolac, diclofenac

- Reversibly inhibit COX-1 and COX-2
- Benefits
  - ↓ pain, redness, swelling (inflammation)
- Adverse effects
  - ↓ platelet aggregation (risk of bleeding)
  - ↓ renal blood flow (ischemia)
  - ↓ GI mucosa (ulcers/bleeding)
  - Interstitial nephritis

Boards&Beyond.

Acute Interstitial Nephritis

- Inflammation of "interstitium"
  - Space between cells
  - Not disease of nephron itself
- Hypersensitivity (allergic) reaction
- Usually triggered by drugs
- Sometimes infections or autoimmune disease
- Classic finding: Urine eosinophils

Boards&Beyond.

Acute Interstitial Nephritis

- Classic presentation
  - Days to weeks after exposure to typical drug
  - Fever, rash
  - Oliguria
  - Increased BUN/Cr
  - Eosinophils in urine

Boards&Beyond.

COX-2 Inhibitors

Celecoxib

- Reversibly inhibit COX-2 only
- Benefits
  - ↓ pain, redness, swelling (inflammation)
  - Less risk GI ulcers/bleeding
- Adverse effects
  - ↑ CV events (MI, stroke) in clinical trials
  - Sulfa drugs (allergy)

Boards&Beyond.

Glucocorticoids

Prednisone, methylprednisolone, hydrocortisone, triamcinolone, dexamethasone, beclomethasone

- Diffuse across cell membranes
- Bind to glucocorticoid receptor (GR)
- GR-steroid complex translocates to nucleus
- Effects via altering gene expression

Boards&Beyond.

Glucocorticoids

Mechanisms of action

- Inactivation NF-KB
  - Key inflammatory transcription factor
  - Mediates response to TNF-α
  - Controls synthesis inflammatory mediators
  - COX-2, PLA2, Lipoxygenase

Boards&Beyond.

Eicosanoids

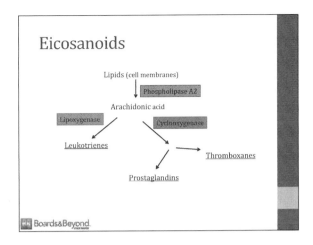

Lipids (cell membranes)

↓ Phospholipase A2

Arachidonic acid

Lipoxygenase | Cyclooxygenase

Leukotrienes

Thromboxanes

Prostaglandins

Glucocorticoids

- Many, many immunosuppressive effects
- Neutrophilic leukocytosis (↑WBCs)
  - Impaired neutrophil migration
- ↓ circulating eosinophils, monocytes, lymphocytes
- ↓ expression many cytokines
  - Interleukins, IFN-γ, TNF-α, GM-CSF

Glucocorticoids
Selected side Effects

- Skin: skin thinning and easy bruising
- Cushingoid appearance/weight gain
  - Truncal obesity, buffalo hump, moon face
- Osteoporosis
- Hyperglycemia
  - ↑ liver gluconeogenesis
  - ↓ glucose uptake fat tissue

Glucocorticoids
Selected side Effects

- Cataracts
- Myopathy (muscle weakness)
  - skeletal muscle catabolism (amino acids) for gluconeogenesis
- Gastritis/peptic ulcers
  - Gastric hyperplasia
  - ↑ acid secretion
  - ↓ mucus synthesis

Avascular Necrosis
Osteonecrosis

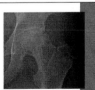

- Bone collapse
- Most commonly femoral head
- Mechanism poorly understood
  - Interruption of blood flow (infract)
  - Demineralization/bone thinning
  - Collapse

Jmarchn/Wikipedia

- Commonly associated with long term steroid use
- Other risk factors:
  - Lupus
  - Sickle cell
  - Alcoholism
  - Trauma

Adrenal Insufficiency

- Long term steroid use suppresses HPA axis
  - Hypothalamus-Pituitary-Adrenal axis
- Abrupt discontinuation → adrenal insufficiency
- Symptoms (adrenal crisis):
  - Dominant feature: Hypotension/shock
  - Anorexia, nausea, vomiting, abdominal pain
  - Weakness, fatigue, lethargy
  - Fever
  - Confusion or coma

Immunosuppressants

Jason Ryan, MD, MPH

Boards&Beyond.

Immune Suppression

- Commonly used drugs:
  - NSAIDs, Steroids
- Less commonly used drugs:
  - Cyclosporine/Tacrolimus
  - Sirolimus
  - Methotrexate
  - Mycophenolate
  - Cyclophosphamide
  - Azathioprine
  - TNF-α inhibitors
  - Hydroxychloroquine

Boards&Beyond.

Cyclosporine & Tacrolimus

- Both drugs inhibit calcineurin
- Calcineurin activates (via dephosphorylation) NFAT
  - Nuclear factor of activated T-cells
  - Important transcription factor for many cytokines

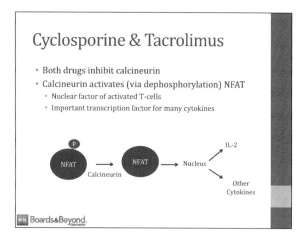

Boards&Beyond.

Cyclosporine & Tacrolimus

- Cyclosporine: binds to cyclophilins
  - Complex inactivates calcineurin
- Tacrolimus: binds to FK-506 binding protein
  - Complex inactivates calcineurin

Boards&Beyond.

Cyclosporine & Tacrolimus

- Autoimmune diseases, organ transplants
- Similar side effects
- Both drugs metabolized P450 system
- Many drug-drug interactions
- Can raise/lower levels/effects

Boards&Beyond.

Cyclosporine & Tacrolimus

- Nephrotoxicity
  - Most important and limiting side effect
  - **Vasoconstriction** of the afferent/efferent arterioles
- Hypertension
  - Via renal vasoconstriction (salt/water retention)
  - Diltiazem drug of choice
  - Impairs cyclosporine metabolism (↑ drug levels)
  - Treats HTN and allows lower dose cyclosporine to be used

Boards&Beyond.

Cyclosporine & Tacrolimus

- Hyperuricemia and gout
- Hyperglycemia (may impair insulin secretion)
- Neurotoxicity (usually tremor)

Cyclosporine

- Two unique side effects
- Not reported with tacrolimus
- Gingival hyperplasia
- Hirsutism

Lesion/Wikipedia

Wikipedia/Public Domain

Sirolimus
Rapamycin

- Kidney transplant, drug-eluting stents
- Inhibits mTOR (mechanistic target of rapamycin)
- Binds FK binding protein
  - Same target as Tacrolimus
  - Does NOT inhibit calcineurin
  - Inhibits mTOR
- Blocks response to IL-2 in B/T cells
  - Blocks signaling pathways
  - Cell cycle arrest in the G1-S phase
  - No growth/proliferation

Sirolimus
Rapamycin

- Anemia, thrombocytopenia, leukopenia
- Hyperlipidemia
  - inhibition of lipoprotein lipase
- Hyperglycemia
  - Insulin resistance

Coronary Stents

- "Drug-eluting stents" (DES)
  - Coated with anti-proliferative drug
  - Blunts scar tissue growth (restenosis)
- Sirolimus
- Everolimus
- Paclitaxel

Wikipedia/Public Domain

Methotrexate

- Chemotherapy, autoimmune diseases
- Mimics folic acid - inhibits dihydrofolate reductase

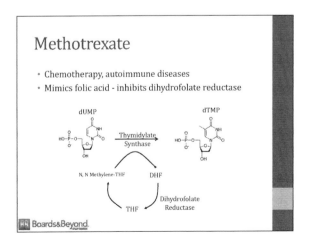

Methotrexate
Side Effects

- Myelosuppression
  - Reversible with leucovorin (folinic acid)
  - Converted to THF
  - Does not require dihydrofolate reductase
  - "Leucovorin rescue"
- Stomatitis/Mucositis (mouth soreness)
  - Occurs with many chemo agents
  - DNA damage → cytokine release
  - Cytokines damage epithelium
  - Loss of mucosal integrity → pain, bacterial growth
- Abnormal LFTs, GI upset

The pathobiology of mucositis. Sonis ST. Nat Rev Cancer. 2004;4(4):277

Mycophenolic acid
CellCept

- Inhibits IMP dehydrogenase
  - Rate-limiting step in purine synthesis in **lymphocytes only**
  - Also, preferentially binds type II isoform IMP dehydrogenase
  - Type II Expressed by **activated lymphocytes**
- ↓ nucleotides → ↓ DNA synthesis in T/B cells
- Bone Marrow Suppression
- GI: Nausea, cramping, abdominal pain

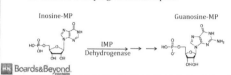

Cyclophosphamide

- Powerful immunosuppressant (also anti-tumor)
- Used in vasculitis, glomerulonephritis (oral)
- Prodrug: Requires bioactivation by liver
  - Converted to phosphoramide mustard
  - Metabolized by P450 system
- "Alkylating agent"
  - Adds an alkyl group to the N7 position
- DNA strands will cross link
- Inhibits DNA replication → cell death

Guanine

Cyclophosphamide
Side Effects

- Myelosuppression
  - ↓WBC, ↓Hct, ↓Plt
- Hemorrhagic cystitis
  - **Acrolein** metabolite toxic to bladder
  - Hematuria +/- dysuria
  - Lower risk with hydration and mesna
  - Mesna: sodium 2-mercaptoethane sulfonate
  - Mesna binds and inactivates acrolein in the urine

Cyclophosphamide
Side Effects

- SIADH
  - Usually IV dosing for chemotherapy
  - **Hyponatremia**; possible **seizures**
  - Compounded by IVF
  - Complex mechanism: More ADH release, less renal response

Azathioprine

- Transplants, autoimmune diseases
- Prodrug converted to 6-Mercaptopurine (6-MP)
  - Analog to hypoxanthine (**purine** like adenine, guanine)
- 6-MP competes for binding to HGPRT
  - Hypoxanthine guanine phosphoribosyltransferase
  - Converts hypoxanthine to inosine monophosphate
  - Also guanine to guanosine monophosphate

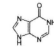 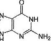 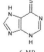

Hypoxanthine   Guanine   6-MP

Azathioprine

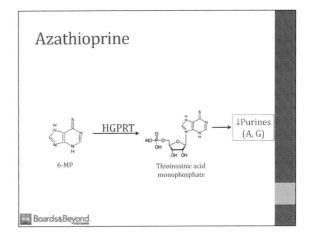

Azathioprine

Azathioprine
Adverse Effects

- Bone marrow suppression
- GI: Anorexia, nausea, and vomiting
- Caution with allopurinol
  - Xanthine oxidase inhibitor
  - Metabolizes purines → uric acid
  - Blunts metabolism of 6-MP/azathioprine
  - ↑ risk of adverse effects

Muromonab-CD3
OKT3

- Monoclonal antibody
- Used in organ transplantation
- Binds to epsilon chain of CD3 (T cells)
- Blocks T-cell activation
- Leads to T-cell depletion from circulation

Muromonab-CD3
OKT3

- Key side effect: **Cytokine release syndrome**
  - Occurs after first or second dose
  - Fevers, rigors, nausea, vomiting, diarrhea, hypotension
  - Sometimes chest pain, dyspnea or wheezing
  - Arthralgias and myalgias
  - Caused by initial activation of T cells → release of cytokines
  - Minimized by pre-medication with steroids, antihistamines

Infliximab

- Antibody against TNF-α
- Used in rheumatoid arthritis, Crohn's
- "Chimeric"
  - Both mouse (murine) and human components
  - Antigen-binding portion of molecule: murine
  - Constant Fc domain: human
- Risk of reactivation TB
  - PPD screening done prior to treatment
- Risk of other infections: bacterial, hepatitis, zoster

Other TNF-α Inhibitors

- Adalimumab (monoclonal antibody TNF-α)
- Golimumab (monoclonal antibody TNF-α)
- Etanercept
  - Made by recombinant DNA
  - Recombinant protein of TNF receptor
  - "Decoy receptor"
  - Binds TNF instead of TNF receptor

Malaria Drugs

- Chloroquine and hydroxychloroquine
- Malaria drugs with immunosuppressive actions
  - Block TLRs in B-cells (↓activation)
  - Weak bases: ↑pH in immune cells → ↓ activity
  - Other actions
- Used in rheumatoid arthritis, SLE

Systemic Lupus Erythematosus

Jason Ryan, MD, MPH

Boards&Beyond

SLE
Systemic Lupus Erythematosus

- Autoimmune disease
- Most patients (90%) are women
- Usually develops age 15 to 45

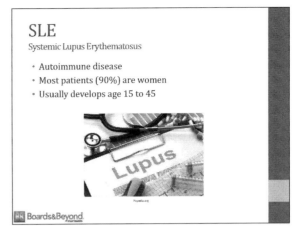

Boards&Beyond

SLE
Systemic Lupus Erythematosus

- Antibodies against nuclear material
  - Key finding: **anti-nuclear antibodies (ANA)**
- Antibody-antigen complexes circulate in plasma
  - **Type III hypersensitivity** reaction
  - Deposit in MANY tissues (diffuse symptoms)
- Antibody-antigen complexes activated complement
  - **Low C3/C4 levels (hypocomplementemia)**
  - Low CH50

Boards&Beyond

SLE
Cause

- Etiology unknown
- Likely genetic, immune, environmental factors
- Viruses and UV light may play a role

Boards&Beyond

Lupus Antibodies

- Anti-nuclear antibodies (ANA)
  - Present in serum of lupus patients
  - Also present in 5% normal patients
  - Also present in many other autoimmune disorders
  - **Sensitive** but not specific
  - Negative test = disease very unlikely
  - Reported as titre: 1:20 or 1:200
  - Often 1:160 considered positive

Boards&Beyond

Lupus Antibodies

- Anti-double stranded DNA (anti-dsDNA)
  - **Specific** for SLE
  - Associated with disease activity (↑ in flares)
  - Associated with renal involvement (glomerulonephritis)
- Anti-smith (anti-Sm)
  - **Specific** for SLE
  - Directed against small nuclear ribonucleoprotein (snRNPs)

Boards&Beyond

snRNPs
Small nuclear ribonucleoprotein

- Combine with RNA transcripts
- Form a "**spliceosome**"
- Removes a portion of the RNA transcript
- Antibodies against RNP (anti-Sm) in lupus

Extractable Nuclear Antigens
ENA Panel

- Panel of blood tests against nuclear antigens

Antibody	Features
Anti-RNP	MCTD, SLE, Scleroderma
Anti-Sm	Specific for Lupus
Anti-SS-A (Ro)	Sjogren's syndrome, SLE, Scleroderma
Anti-SS-B (La)	Sjogren's syndrome, SLE, Scleroderma
Scl-70	Specific for scleroderma
Anti-Jo-1	Polymyositis

SLE
Symptoms

- **Flares** and remissions common
- Fever, weight loss, fatigue, lymphadenopathy

Malar Rash

- Classic lupus skin finding
- "Butterfly" rash
- Common on **sunlight** exposure
- Can also see **"discoid" lesion**
  - Circular skin lesion
  - Classically on forearm

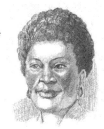

Wikipedia/Public Domain

Raynaud Phenomenon

- White/blue fingertips
- Painful on exposure to cold
- Vasospasm of the artery → ischemia
- Can lead to fingertip ulcers
- Seen in other conditions
  - Isolated
  - Other autoimmune disorders

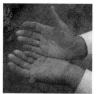

Jamclaassen~commonswiki /Wikipedia

SLE
Symptoms

- Oral or nasal ulcers
- Arthritis (tender, swollen joints)
- Serositis

de:Benutzer:Padawan/Wikipedia

  - Inflammation of pleura (pain with inspiration)
  - Inflammation of pericardium (pericarditis)
- "Penias"
  - Anemia, thrombocytopenia, leukopenia
  - Antibody attack of cells (Type II hypersensitivity)

Database Center for Life Science (DBCLS)

Lupus Cerebritis
CNS Involvement

- Cognitive dysfunction
  - Confusion
  - Memory loss
- Stroke
- Seizures

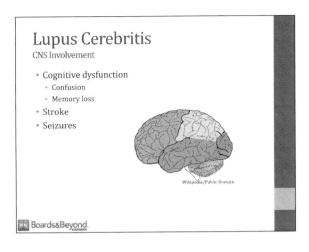

Wikipedia/Public Domain

Boards&Beyond

Lupus Nephropathy

- Nephritic or nephrotic syndrome (or both)
- Common cause of death in lupus
- **Diffuse proliferative glomerular nephritis**
  - Most common SLE renal syndrome
  - Nephritic syndrome
- **Membranous glomerular nephritis**
  - Nephrotic syndrome

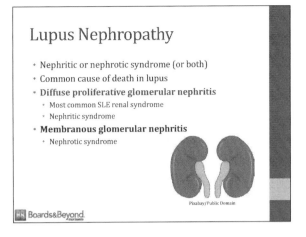

Pixabay/Public Domain

Boards&Beyond

Cardiac Manifestations

- Libman-Sacks (marantic) endocarditis
- Nonbacterial inflammation of valves
- Classically affects **both sides** of mitral valve

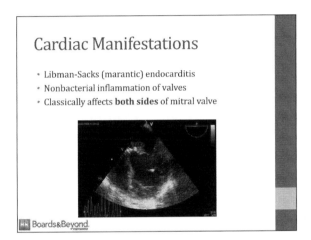

Boards&Beyond

Anti-Phospholipid Antibodies

- Occur in association with lupus
  - Can also occur as a primary problem
- Antibodies against proteins in phospholipids
- Three important clinical consequences
  - "Antiphospholipid syndrome"
  - Increased risk of venous and **arterial thrombosis**
  - DVT, stroke, fetal loss
  - **Increased PTT**
  - **False positive** syphilis (RPR/VDRL)

Boards&Beyond

Anti-Phospholipid Antibodies

- **Anti-cardiolipin**
  - False positive RPR/VDRL
  - Syphilis also produces these antibodies
- **"Lupus anticoagulant"**
  - Interferes with PTT test
  - False elevation
- **Anti-β2 glycoprotein**

Boards&Beyond

SLE
Diagnosis

- Need four of 11 criteria

1. Malar Rash	2. Discoid Rash
3. Photosensitivity	4. Oral ulcers
5. Arthritis	6. Serositis
7. Cerebritis	8. Renal disease
9. "Penias"	10. ANA
11. Anti-dsDNA or Anti-Sm or anti-phospholipid	

Boards&Beyond

59

Drug-Induced Lupus

- Lupus-like syndrome after taking a drug
- Classic drugs: **INH, hydralazine, procainamide**
- Often rash, arthritis, penias, ANA+
- Kidney or CNS involvement rare
- Key features: anti-histone antibodies
- Resolves on stopping the drug

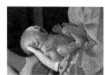

Pixabay/Public Domain

SLE
Treatment

- Steroids
- Other immunosuppressants
- Avoid sunlight
  - Many patients photosensitive
  - Can trigger flares
- Causes of death
  - Renal failure
  - Infection (immunosuppression drugs)
  - Coronary disease (SLE → increased risk)

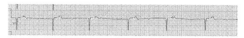

Pixabay/Public Domain

Neonatal Lupus

- Maternal antibodies → fetus
- 1 to 2% babies born if maternal autoimmune disease
  - Systemic lupus erythematosus
  - **Sjogren's syndrome**
  - +SSA/Ro or + SSB/La – either disease

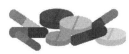

Ernest F/Wikipedia

Neonatal Lupus

- At birth or first few weeks of life
- **Rash**
  - Multiple red, circular lesions on face, scalp
- **Congenital complete heart block**
  - Slow heart rate (50s)
  - Often does not respond to steroids

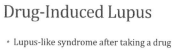

Rheumatoid Arthritis

Rheumatoid Arthritis

Jason Ryan, MD, MPH

Rheumatoid Arthritis

- Autoimmune disorder
- Inflammation of joints especially hands, wrists
- More common in women
- Usual age of onset 40 - 60

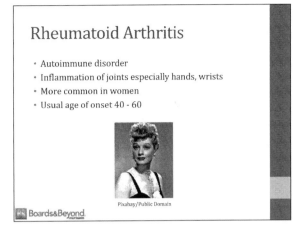

Pixabay/Public Domain

Rheumatoid Arthritis

- **Synovium**
  - Thin layer of tissue (few cells thick)
  - Lines joints and tendon sheaths
  - Secretes **hyaluronic acid** to lubricate joint space
- **Inflammation**
  - Unknown trigger
  - Overproduction of TNF and IL-6

Rheumatoid Arthritis

- **Synovial hypertrophy**
  - Thickens into **pannus**
  - Infiltrated with inflammatory cells, granulation tissue
  - Increase in synovial fluid
  - Erodes into cartilage, bone
- Antibody-mediated
  - **Type III hypersensitivity**

Synovial Joint

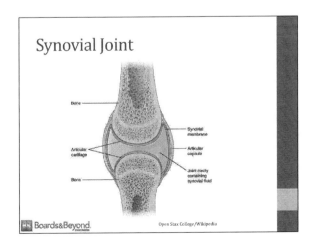

Open Stax College/Wikipedia

Rheumatoid Arthritis

- **Symmetric** joint inflammation
- Gradual onset
- Pain, stiffness, swelling
- Classically "**morning stiffness**"
  - Joint stiffness >1 hour after rising
  - Improves with use
- May have systemic symptoms (fever)

Rheumatoid Arthritis

* Classically affects **MCP and PIP** joints of hands
  * Often tender to touch
* DIP joints spared

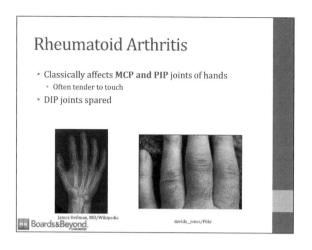

James Heilman, MD/Wikipedia

davida_jones/Flikr

Rheumatoid Arthritis

* Bones can erode/deviate
* **Ulnar deviation**
  * Swelling of MCP joints → deviated wrist
* **Swan neck deformity**
  * Hyperextended PIP joint
  * Flexed DIP

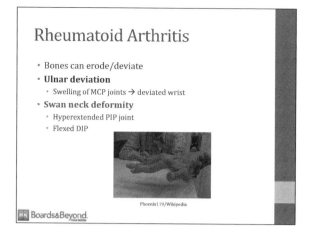

Phoenix119/Wikipedia

Rheumatoid Arthritis

* Other joints:
  * Wrists
  * Elbows
  * Knees
  * Hips
  * Toes

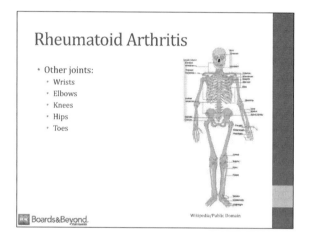

Wikipedia/Public Domain

Rheumatoid Arthritis

* Baker's cyst (popliteal cyst)
  * Synovium-lined sac at back of knee
  * Continuous with the joint space
  * If ruptures → symptoms similar to DVT

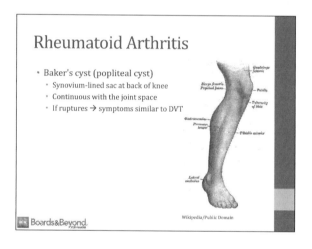

Wikipedia/Public Domain

Rheumatoid Arthritis

* Serositis
  * **Pleuritis**, pleural effusion
  * **Pericarditis**, pericardial effusion

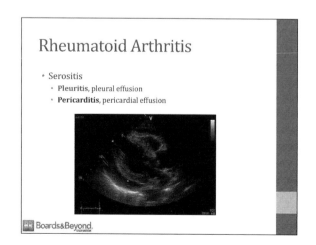

Subcutaneous nodules

* Palpable nodules common (20 to 35% patients)
* Almost always occur in patients with RF+
* Common on elbow (can occur anywhere)
* Central necrosis surrounded by macrophages/lymphocytes
* Usually no specific treatment

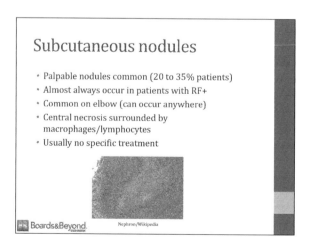

Nephron/Wikipedia

Rheumatoid Arthritis

- Episcleritis
  - Red, painful without discharge
- Scleritis
  - Often bilateral
  - Dark, red eyes
  - Deep ocular pain on eye movement
- Uveitis
  - Anterior/posterior
  - Floaters if posterior

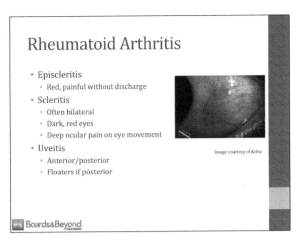

Image courtesy of Kribz

Sjogren's Syndrome

- Salivary and lacrimal glands
- Dry eyes, dry mouth (sicca symptoms)
- Commonly associated with rheumatoid arthritis

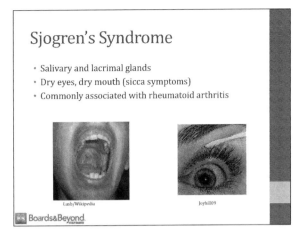

Lusb/Wikipedia   Joyhill09

Osteoporosis

- Accelerated by RA
- Also often worsened by steroid treatment
- 30 percent ↑risk of major fracture
- 40 percent ↑risk hip fracture

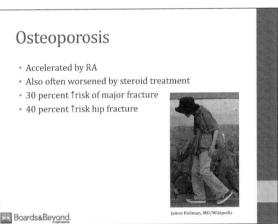

James Heilman, MD/Wikipedia

Rheumatoid Arthritis

- ~80% positive rheumatoid factor
  - Antibodies against Fc portion of IgG antibody
  - "Seropositive" rheumatoid arthritis
  - Poor specificity
  - Positive in endocarditis, Hep B, Hep C
  - Positive in Sjogren's, Lupus
- Antibodies to **citrullinated peptides** (ACPA)
  - Specific marker of RA

Urea Cycle

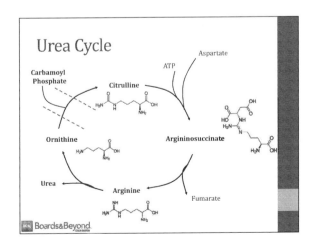

Citrulline

- Non-standard amino acid - not encoded by genome
- Incorporated into proteins via post-translational modification
- More incorporation in inflammation
- Anti-citrulline peptide antibodies used in RA
  - Up to 80% of patients with RA

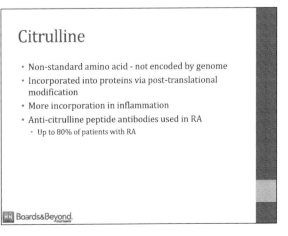

Rheumatoid Arthritis

- Elevated **CRP and ESR**
- Strong association with **HLA-DR4**

Treatment

- NSAIDs
- Steroids
- Disease-modifying antirheumatic drugs (DMARDs)
  - Protect joints from destruction
  - Methotrexate
  - Azathioprine
  - Cyclosporine
  - Hydroxychloroquine
  - Sulfasalazine
  - Leflunomide
  - TNF-a inhibitors (antibodies against TNF-α)

Sulfasalazine

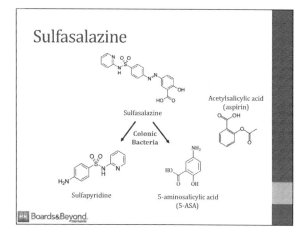

Leflunomide

- Inhibits dihydroorotate dehydrogenase
- Inhibits **pyrimidine** synthesis
- Side effects: diarrhea, abnormal LFTs, ↓WBCs
- Also used in psoriatic arthritis

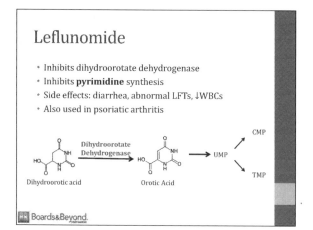

Infliximab

- Antibody against **TNF-α**
- Used in rheumatoid arthritis, Crohn's
- Risk of **reactivation TB**
  - **PPD screening** done prior to treatment
- Risk of other infections: bacterial, zoster

Other TNF-α Inhibitors

- Adalimumab (monoclonal antibody TNF-α)
- Golimumab (monoclonal antibody TNF-α)
- Etanercept
  - Recombinant protein of TNF receptor
  - "Decoy receptor"
  - Binds TNF instead of TNF receptor

Long Term Complications

- Increased risk of **coronary disease**
  - Leading cause of mortality
- **Amyloidosis**
  - Secondary (AA) amyloidosis

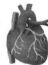

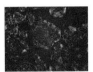

Ed Uthman, MD/Wikipedia

Boards&Beyond.

Felty Syndrome

- Syndrome of **splenomegaly**, **neutropenia** in RA
- Classically occurs many years after onset RA
- Usually in patient with severe RA
  - Joint deformity
  - Extra-articular disease
- Improves with RA therapy

Bob Blaylock/Wikipedia

Wikipedia/Public Domain

Boards&Beyond.

Scleroderma

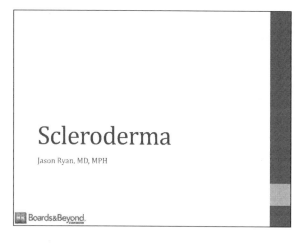

Scleroderma
Jason Ryan, MD, MPH

Scleroderma
Systemic Sclerosis

- Autoimmune disorder
- Stiff, hardened tissue (sclerosis)
- Skin, other organ systems involved

Scleroderma
Systemic Sclerosis

- Endothelial cell damage
  - Trigger unclear
  - Antibodies, cytokines → damage
- Result is **fibroblast** activation
- **Excess collagen** deposition

Scleroderma
Systemic Sclerosis

- Most common demographic is **women**
- Peak onset **30-50 years old**
- Presents in two clinical syndromes
  - Diffuse
  - Limited (CREST)

Diffuse Scleroderma

- Diffuse **skin thickening**
- **Raynaud's phenomenon**
  - Often initial sign
  - Followed ~ 1 year with other signs/symptoms
- Early involvement of visceral organs
  - Renal disease – renal failure
  - GI tract – dysmotility, heartburn
  - Heart: pericarditis, myocarditis, conduction disease
  - Joints/muscles: Arthralgia, myalgias

Pulmonary Disease

- Pulmonary hypertension
  - Can progress to right heart failure
  - RV heave
  - Elevated jugular veins
  - Pitting edema
  - Routine monitoring: echocardiography
- Interstitial lung disease

Scleroderma Renal Crisis

* Life-threatening complication of diffuse scleroderma
* Acute worsening of renal function
* Marked hypertension
* Responds to **ACE inhibitors**

Limited Scleroderma
CREST

* "Limited" skin involvement
  * Skin sclerosis restricted to hands
  * Sometimes distal forearm, face or neck
* CREST
  * Calcinosis
  * Raynaud's phenomenon
  * Esophageal dysmotility
  * Sclerodactyly
  * Telangiectasias

Calcinosis
CREST

* Calcium deposits in subcutaneous tissue
* Bumps on **elbows, knees and fingers**
* Can break skin, **leak** white liquid
* **X-rays** of hands may show soft tissue calcifications

Raynaud's Phenomenon
CREST

* White/blue fingertips
* Painful on exposure to cold
* Vasospasm of the artery → ischemia
* Can lead to fingertip ulcers
* Often 1st sign for **years/decades**
* Seen in other conditions
  * Isolated
  * Other autoimmune disorders

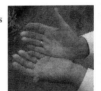

Jamclaassen~commonswiki /Wikipedia

Esophageal Dysmotility
CREST

* Difficulty swallowing
  * Dysmotility
* Reflux/heartburn
  * LES **hypotonia**
  * "Incompetent LES"

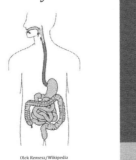

Olek Remesz/Wikipedia

Sclerodactyly
CREST

* Fibrosis of skin of hands
* Can begin as fingers puffy, hard to bend
* Later, skin often be becomes **shiny** skin
* **Thickened skin** (can't pinch the skin)
* **Loss of wrinkles**
* Severe form: hands like claws
* Also seen in diffuse type

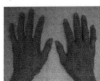

James Heilman /Wikipedia

Telangiectasias
CREST

- Skin lesions
- Dilated capillaries
- **Face**, hands, mucous membranes

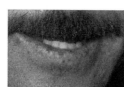

Herbert L. Fred, MD and Hendrik A. van Dijk

Boards&Beyond.

Limited Scleroderma
CREST

- Generally more benign course than diffuse
    - Rarely involves heart, kidneys
- Main risk is **pulmonary disease**
- Leading cause of death
- Pulmonary hypertension
- Interstitial lung disease
- Similar features to diffuse scleroderma

Boards&Beyond.

Scleroderma
Systemic Sclerosis

- Antinuclear antibody (ANA) – Not specific
- **Anti-topoisomerase I (anti-Scl-70) antibody**
    - Diffuse disease
- **Anti-centromere antibody (ACA)**
    - Limited disease
    - CREST = centromere
- **Anti-RNA polymerase III antibody**
    - Diffuse disease
    - Associated with rapidly progressive skin involvement
    - Also increased risk for renal crisis

Boards&Beyond.

Scleroderma
Systemic Sclerosis

- Treatment usually aimed at organ system
    - GI tract: proton pump inhibitors
    - Raynaud's: Calcium channel blockers
    - Pulmonary: Pulmonary hypertension drugs
- Immunosuppressants have limited role
    - Little proven benefit
    - Used in rare, special cases

Boards&Beyond.

Primary Biliary Cirrhosis

- T-cell destruction small bile ducts
- Often presents jaundice, fatigue, **itching**
- Can lead to cirrhosis and liver failure
- Elevated conjugated bilirubin, alkaline phosphatase
- Associated with scleroderma
    - 5 to 15% PBC patients have **limited scleroderma**
- Also associated with **Sjogren's**, Lupus, RA
- Also Hashimoto's thyroiditis

Boards&Beyond.

Sjogren's Syndrome

Jason Ryan, MD, MPH

Sjogren's Syndrome

- Autoimmune disorder
- Destruction of salivary and lacrimal glands

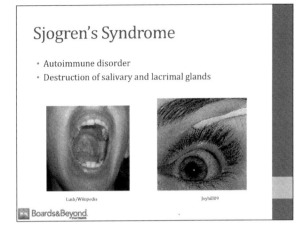

Lusb/Wikipedia   Joyhill09

Sjogren's Syndrome

- Dry eyes (keratoconjunctivitis sicca)
  - May present as feeling of dirt/debris in eyes
- Dry mouth (xerostomia)
  - Difficulty chewing dry foods (i.e. crackers)
  - Cavities
  - Bad breath

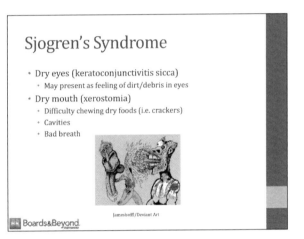

Jamesbrdfl/Deviant Art

Sjogren's Syndrome
"Extraglandular" disease symptoms

- Xerosis
  - Dry, scaly skin
  - Often lower extremities and axilla
- Joints: **arthralgias** or arthritis
- **Raynaud's** phenomena
- Many, many other potential symptoms

Sjogren's Syndrome

- More common among women
- Age of onset usually in 40s
- Many elderly patients have "sicca symptoms"
  - Dry mouth, dry eyes
  - Not due to Sjogren's
  - Antibody tests and/or biopsy = normal

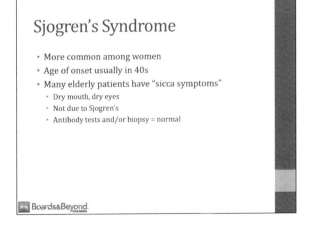

Sjogren's Syndrome

- Lymphocyte mediated
  - Type IV hypersensitivity disorder
  - Biopsy of salivary gland: **Lymphocytic sialadenitis**

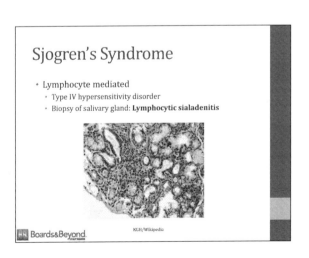

KGH/Wikipedia

Sjogren's Syndrome

- Primary or secondary
  - Often associated with **rheumatoid arthritis** and **lupus**
  - 40-65% of primary biliary cirrhosis patients have Sjögren's

Antibodies

- Four relevant antibody tests

Antinuclear antibody (ANA)	Not specific
Rheumatoid Factor	Seen in 1° and 2°
Anti-SS-A (Ro)	Associated with neonatal lupus
Anti-SS-B (La)	Associated with neonatal lupus

Schirmer Test

- Tests reflex tear production
- Filter paper placed near lower eyelid
- Patient closes eyes
- Amount of wetting (mm) measured over 5 minutes

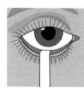

Jmarchn/Wikipedia

Salivary Testing

- Salivary gland scintigraphy
  - Nuclear test
  - Low uptake of radionuclide in patients with SS
- Whole sialometry
  - Measurement of saliva production
  - Patient collects all saliva over 15 minutes
  - Sample weighed

Diagnosis

- Any 4 of 6 criteria
- Must include either histopathology or autoantibodies

Eye symptoms
Oral symptoms
Ocular Signs (Schirmer test)
Oral signs (Salivary testing)
Biopsy: Lymphocytic sialadenitis
Anti-SSa or Anti-SSb

Treatment

- Good oral hygiene
- Artificial saliva
- Muscarinic agonists: **pilocarpine**
- Sometimes steroids for extraglandular disease

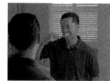

Bill Branson/Public Domain

B cell Lymphoma

- Increased risk among Sjogren's patients
  - 5-10% of patients
- May present as persistent **unilateral swollen gland**
  - May mimic past swelling

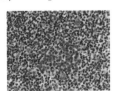

KGH/Wikipedia

Neonatal Lupus

- Maternal antibodies → fetus
- 1 to 2% babies born if maternal autoimmune disease
  - Systemic lupus erythematosus
  - Sjögren's syndrome
  - +SSA/Ro or + SSB/La – either disease

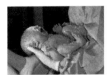

Ernest F/Wikipedia

Neonatal Lupus

- At birth or first few weeks of life
- **Rash**
  - Multiple red, circular lesions on face, scalp
- **Congenital complete heart block**
  - Slow heart rate (50s)
  - Often does not respond to steroids

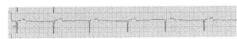

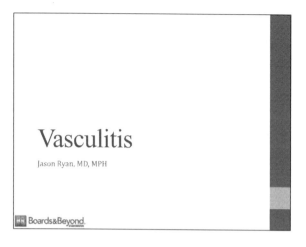

Vasculitis

* Inflammation of blood vessels
* Leukocytes in blood vessel walls
* Typical inflammation symptoms
  * Fever
  * Myalgias
  * Arthralgias
  * Fatigue
* Organ/disease specific symptoms
  * Vessel lumen narrows or occludes from inflammation

Classification

Vessel Type	Diseases
Large	Temporal Arteritis Takayasu's Arteritis
Medium	Polyarteritis Nodosa Kawasaki Disease Buerger's disease
Small	Churg-Strauss Wegener's granulomatosis Microscopic polyangiitis Henoch-Schönlein purpura

Palpable Purpura

* Purpura: red-purple skin lesions
* Extravagation of blood into the skin
* Does not blanch when pressed

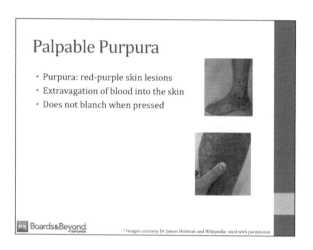

* Images courtesy Dr. James Heilman and Wikipedia; used with permission

Palpable Purpura

* Non-palpable purpura
  * Usually non-inflammatory
  * Petechiae (small), Ecchymosis (large)
* Palpable purpura
  * Occurs in vasculitis
  * Raised
  * Small vessel inflammation
  * Leukocytoclastic vasculitis

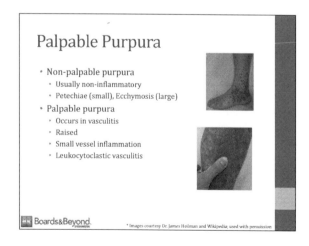

* Images courtesy Dr. James Heilman and Wikipedia; used with permission

Vasculitis Treatment

* Most treated with **steroids or cyclophosphamide**

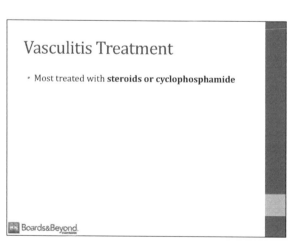

Classification

Vessel	Diseases	Features
Large	Temporal Arteritis Takayasu's Arteritis	Elderly female, headache Asian female, pulseless
Medium	Kawasaki Disease Buerger's disease Polyarteritis Nodosa	Asian child, red rash, tongue Smoker's hands Hep B
Small	Henoch-Schönlein purpura Churg-Strauss Wegener's granulomatosis Microscopic polyangiitis	Child, URI, melena Asthma, eosinophils, p-ANCA Sinus, kidneys, lungs, c-ANCA Kidneys, lungs, p-ANCA

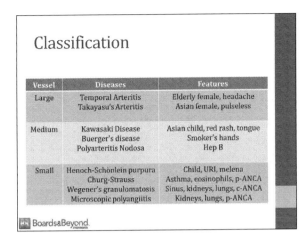

Large Vessel Vasculitis

- Temporal arteritis
- Takayasu's arteritis
- Granulomatous inflammation
- Narrowing of large arteries

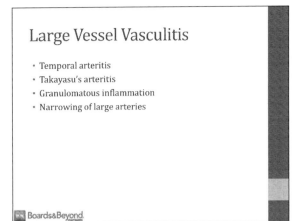

Temporal Arteritis
Giant Cell Arteritis

- Narrowing of temporal artery system
- Headache, jaw claudication (pain on chewing)
- If not treated → blindness
  - Ophthalmic artery occlusion

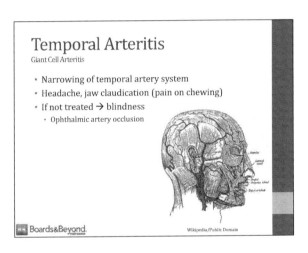

Wikipedia/Public Domain

Temporal Arteritis
Giant Cell Arteritis

- High ESR
- Diagnosis: Biopsy temporal artery (granulomas)
- Treat with high dose steroids (don't wait for biopsy)
- Classic case:
  - Elderly female with headache
  - Pain on chewing
  - High ESR

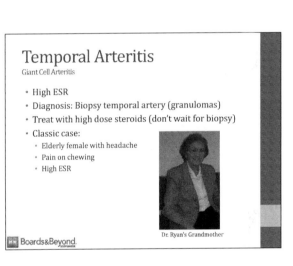

Dr. Ryan's Grandmother

Takayasu's Arteritis

- Granulomatous thickening of aortic arch and branches
- Up to 90% of cases occur in women
- Greatest prevalence in Asia

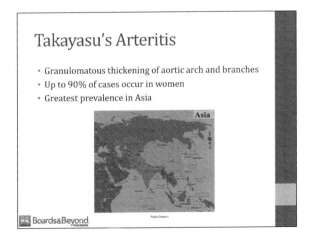

Public Domain

Takayasu's Arteritis

- Classic symptoms: Weak pulses one arm
- "Pulseless disease"
  - Proximal great vessels
  - BP difference between arms/legs
  - Bruits over arteries
- ↑ESR
- Treat with steroids

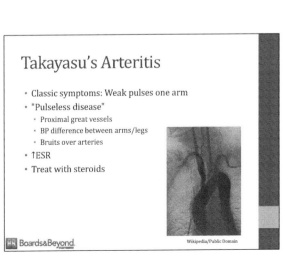

Wikipedia/Public Domain

Kawasaki Disease

- Autoimmune attack of medium vessels
- Most cases occur in children
- Classic involvement: **skin, lips, tongue**
  - Diffuse, red rash
  - Palms, soles → later desquamates
  - Changes in lips/oral mucosa: "**strawberry tongue**"
- Feared complication: coronary aneurysms
  - Rupture → myocardial infarction
- Treatment: IV immunoglobulin and aspirin

AHA Scientific Statement: Diagnosis, Treatment, and Long-Term Management of Kawasaki Disease.
Circulation 2004;110:2747-2771

Boards&Beyond.

Kawasaki Disease

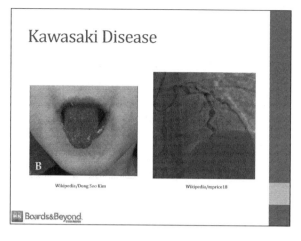

Wikipedia/Dong Soo Kim   Wikipedia/mprice18

Boards&Beyond.

Kawasaki Disease

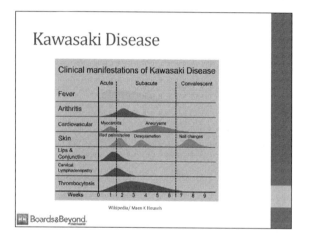

Wikipedia/ Maen K Househ

Boards&Beyond.

Scarlet Fever

- Fever, sore throat, diffuse red rash
- Many small papules ("sandpaper" skin)
- Classic finding: Strawberry tongue
- Eventually skin desquamates

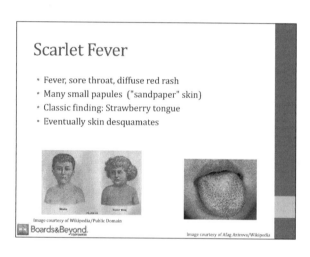

Image courtesy of Wikipedia/Public Domain

Image courtesy of Afag Azirova/Wikipedia

Boards&Beyond.

Reye's Syndrome

- Encephalopathy, liver failure, fatty infiltration
- Symptoms: vomiting, confusion, seizures, coma
- Often follows viral illness
  - Influenza, varicella
- Caused by diffuse mitochondrial insult
- Associated with aspirin use in children
  - Generally, aspirin not used for kids
- Only exception is Kawasaki

Boards&Beyond.

Buerger's Disease
thromboangiitis obliterans

- Male smokers
- Poor blood flow to hands/feet
  - Gangrene
  - Autoamputation of digits
  - Superficial nodular phlebitis
    - Tender nodules over course of a vein
- Raynaud's phenomenon
- Segmental thrombosing vasculitis
- Treatment: Smoking cessation

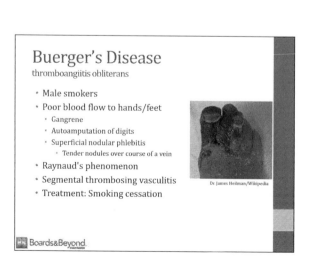

Dr. James Heilman/Wikipedia

Boards&Beyond.

Polyarteritis Nodosa

- **Immune complex mediated** disease: medium vessels
  - Type III hypersensitivity reactions
- Classic demographic: Hep B+
- Nerves: Motor/sensory deficits
- Skin: Nodules, purpura
- Kidneys: Renal failure

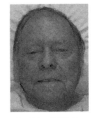

James Heilman, MD/Wikipedia

James Heilman, MD/Wikipedia

Polyarteritis Nodosa

- Many aneurysms and constrictions on arteriogram
  - Kidney, liver, and mesenteric arteries
  - Rosary sign
- Transmural inflammation of medium vessel wall
  - Fibrinoid necrosis

Polyarteritis Nodosa

- Classic case:
  - Hep B+, nerve defects, skin nodules, purpura, renal failure
- Diagnosis:
  - Angiogram (aneurysms)
  - Tissue biopsy of affected system
- Treatment: Corticosteroids, cyclophosphamide

Wikipedia/mprice18

Henoch-Schonlein purpura

- Most common childhood systemic vasculitis
- Often follows URI
- Associated with **IgA**
  - Vasculitis from IgA complex deposition
  - IgA nephropathy
- Also C3 deposition

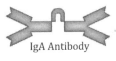

IgA Antibody

Martin Brändli /Wikipedia

Henoch-Schonlein purpura

- Skin: palpable purpura on buttocks/legs
- GI: abdominal pain, melena
- Kidney: Nephritis

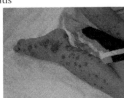

Public Domain/Wikipedia

Henoch-Schonlein purpura

- Classic case:
  - Child with recent URI
  - Palpable purpura
  - Melena
- Tissue biopsy is best test
- Usually self-limited
- Feared result: renal failure
  - More common adults
- Severe cases: steroids/cyclophosphamide (rarely done)

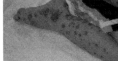

Emmanuelm/Wikipedia

ANCA Diseases
Anti-neutrophil cytoplasmic antibodies

- Churg-Strauss syndrome
- Wegener's Granulomatosis
- Microscopic Polyangiitis
- All have pulmonary involvement
- All have renal involvement
  - Crescentic RPGN
  - "Pauci-immune"
  - Paucity of Ig (negative IF)
  - Nephritic syndrome
  - Proteinuria, hematuria

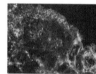

Daisuke Koya, Kazuyuki Shibuya, Ryuichi Kikkawa and Masakazu Haneda.

Images courtesy of bilalbanday

ANCA Diseases
Anti-neutrophil cytoplasmic antibodies

- ANCA
  - Autoantibodies
  - Attack neutrophil proteins
- Two patterns distinguish diseases
- c-ANCA (cytoplasmic)
  - Usually proteinase 3 (PR3) antibodies
  - Wegener's only
- p-ANCA (perinuclear)
  - Usually myeloperoxidase (MPO) antibodies
  - Churg-Strauss and Microscopic Polyangiitis

Dr Graham Beards/Wikipedia

Churg-Strauss syndrome

- Asthma, sinusitis, neuropathy
- Eosinophilia
- p-ANCA, elevated IgE level
- Palpable purpura
- Granulomatous, necrotizing vasculitis
- Can also involve heart, GI, kidneys
- Treatment: steroids, cyclophosphamide

Bobjgalindo/Wikipedia

Wegener's Granulomatosis
(granulomatosis with polyangiitis)

- Sinusitis, otitis media, hemoptysis
  - Upper and lower airway disease
- Renal: hematuria, red cell casts
- Purpura
- Granulomas on biopsy
- c-ANCA
- Treatment: steroids, cyclophosphamide

BruceBlaus/Wikipedia

Microscopic Polyangiitis

- Hemoptysis, kidney failure, purpura
- Just like Wegner's except
  - No upper airway disease (sinusitis)
  - p-ANCA not c-ANCA
  - No granulomas on biopsy
- Treatment: steroids and cyclophosphamide

Goodpasture's Syndrome

- Antibody to collagen (type II hypersensitivity)
  - Antibodies to alpha-3 chain of type IV collagen
  - Anti-GBM
  - Anti-alveoli
- Hemoptysis and nephritic syndrome
- Linear IF (IgG, C3)
- Classic case
  - Young adult
  - Male
  - Hemoptysis
  - Hematuria

Images courtesy of bilalbanday

Treatment Summary

Diseases	Treatment
Temporal Arteritis	Steroids
Takayasu's Arteritis	Steroids
Polyarteritis Nodosa	Steroids/CycP
Kawasaki Disease	IVIG/Aspirin
Buerger's disease	Smoking Cessation
Churg-Strauss	Steroids/CycP
Wegener's granulomatosis	Steroids/CycP
Microscopic polyangiitis	Steroids/CycP
Henoch-Schönlein purpura	Steroids/CycP

Blood Test Summary

Diseases	Test
Temporal Arteritis	↑ESR
Takayasu's Arteritis	↑ESR
Kawasaki Disease	--
Buerger's disease	--
Polyarteritis Nodosa	--
Henoch-Schönlein purpura	--
Churg-Strauss	p-ANCA/IgE
Wegener's granulomatosis	c-ANCA
Microscopic polyangiitis	p-ANCA